CHALLENGING THE YEARS

Challenging the Years

Yoga Wisdom and Modern Knowledge for Healthier and Longer Life

MICHAEL VOLIN

1817

HARPER & ROW, PUBLISHERS
NEW YORK
HAGERSTOWN
SAN FRANCISCO
LONDON

I wish to dedicate this book
to my students on five continents
who are challenging the years using
methods described in this book.

Acknowledgments: I would like to thank Barbara Knott for editing the manuscript and Charles Knott for taking the photographs.

I would also like to thank my students who posed for the illustrations in this book.

FIRST EDITION

Designed by Sidney Feinberg

Library of Congress Cataloging in Publication Data

Volin, Michael.
    Challenging the years.
    Includes index.
    1. Yoga, Hatha. 2. Hygiene, Oriental.
3. Health. 4. Rejuvenation. 5. Longevity.
I. Title.
RA781.7.V57   613.7   78–69624
ISBN 0–06–014469–6

---

79 80 81 82 83 10 9 8 7 6 5 4 3 2 1

Contents

Preface

The first step toward rejuvenation is to understand the difference between the chronological and the physiological ages of the human body. We cannot change our date of birth, but we can alter our physiological age, which refers to the condition of our bodies. In fact, there is nothing magical in reversing the biological clock. Ancient yoga and modern science finally agree that the body is capable of rejuvenation. By adjusting weight, reshaping the body, regaining flexibility, and improving muscle tone, blood circulation, digestion, elimination, and metabolism, we can literally grow younger.

By learning the methods presented in this book—correct breathing, relaxation, constructive mental habits—any dedicated student can prolong the creative part of his life by twenty years; in many cases, one can reverse aging processes that have already set in. It is important to remember that rejuvenation is not an overnight miracle. It requires physical, mental, and spiritual disciplines that must be built up gradually to have a lasting effect. Six to nine months of daily exercises, diet, breathing practices, and meditations will begin to show positive results.

In this book I will share with the reader the experiences

and the knowledge that I acquired in the ashrams of China, Tibet, and India. Yogic methods practiced in these countries were given to me in the traditional *mouth-to-ear*[1] way, and some techniques for delaying aging, to the best of my knowledge, have never been revealed to the Western world.

During almost fifty years of teaching yoga in the East and West, I have had many students experience rebirth both physically and spiritually. Surely that is the most remarkable experience of a lifetime. Older people, as they reach their sixties and seventies, often feel that their lives are approaching the end of a gray tunnel and that there is no light ahead, only the sensation of the inevitability of the end. To be reborn means that they are suddenly aware of the tunnel opening again into a vast light full of new and continuous life experiences, and that they are acquiring a certain mastery over the passage of time. For these people, life literally starts anew. Young people who regularly practice the techniques presented in this book can prolong their youth into what is now considered the middle years of life. Middle-aged people can slough off any manifestations of premature aging by getting back in touch with their youthful selves and prolonging their creative years.

---

1. Some of the techniques in ashrams of the East are kept in secret and literally passed from teacher to student by whispering into the ear, hence the expression "mouth-to-ear" tradition.

Introduction

Many years ago in China my Taoist teacher, to test
my inner strength and my willingness to further my studies, sent me to a remote ashram. Following tradition, I
walked all the way, begging for food and refusing any
kind of transportation. The distance from my home to
the ashram was about 300 miles through rough and wild
parts of China infested by runaway soldiers who had
turned into bandits. During the two months that it took
me to complete the journey, I almost lost my life on two
occasions. Once, for over a week, I was marooned beside
a flooded river without food. Later I was caught by bandits who kept me for several days in a pit. It took all
my eloquence and perseverance to talk them into setting
me free without cropping my ears, which they threatened
to do if a ransom were not paid. In fact, I was so persuasive
that the head of the band provided me with an escort
the rest of the way to my destination. He told me that
the next region was controlled by his brother, who was
not as kind as he, and that his brother would surely chop
off my head together with my ears unless I were protected. With his help, I arrived at my destination, much
thinner and a lot wiser than when I started on the journey.
There I was admitted into the ashram and settled into

a corner of the community room, which became my home for the next several months.

After days of quiet waiting (things were not rushed in China), I inquired very humbly about the master. I was told that he was not available. I could hardly conceal my disappointment. Kindly brothers, knowing the story of my quest, said that I could wait until the master returned. They finally volunteered, rather casually, an explanation for his absence: "He's growing a new body." They said that he would be only too glad to see me when the time came.

I settled down to wait and, in the meantime, fell into the strict routine of the monastery, where time passed uneventfully until the unforgettable arrival of the master. The kind, all-knowing eyes of a sage looked out of an ageless, strangely immobile face. He was slender, of middle height, and his skin looked remarkably youthful, as if untouched by time. He looked hardly more than forty, yet I was told that he was well over ninety when he started rejuvenation.

For a time, he moved in silence, slowly and with deliberation, as he passed among us in the ashram. Finally, he began to take more notice of the events around him. His eyes stopped at me more and more often. One morning he gestured to me to come closer. "Little brother, I learned all about you," he said, smiling. "Sit down with me for a while." We experienced a sensation of great mutual rapport, and I felt great joy when he accepted me as a student.

As I look back, I think now that my encounter with this master was perhaps the greatest experience of my life. I may have been the first Westerner to witness the remarkable result of one person's "growing a new body." I was in my twenties at the time and in excellent physical condition. At that stage I did not need a new body. Nevertheless, I made a point to learn as much as possible about this master's mysterious methods, as well as many techniques of Chinese yoga related to controlling the aging process. This branch of yoga emphasized longevity, reverence for old age, and the nurturing of a long, healthy, and creative winter of life. Later, spending time in ashrams throughout remote parts of China, Tibet, and India, I had opportunities to learn many yoga practices designed to gain mastery over time.

Chinese or Taoist yoga, in particular, contains an esoteric tradition which embraces fragments of several yogas. The highest aim of this yoga, which has no definitive name, is to overcome the laws of karma and incarnation and to attain immortality even of the physical body—in other words, to become avataras (a Sanskrit name for an incarnation of a divine being). The secret doctrines of this yoga contain many techniques that can arrest the aging processes of the body.

Traditional scriptures of the East allude to at least eighty different methods of rejuvenation. Some of these methods have been lost forever; others, such as herbal rejuvenation, are little known in the Western world. At present, nearly intact prescriptions for retarding age survive in various schools of yoga. However, some of the most effective techniques have been kept secret, passed only to chosen disciples in the mouth-to-ear custom of remote ashrams and monasteries of the East. A careful selection of these age-delaying and rejuvenating methods suitable for Western students are presented in this book.

In my own teaching I have often spoken of a particular blending of yogic techniques designed to slow down the aging process as "avatara yoga." This designation will not be found in scholarly treatises on yoga, ancient or modern. In the tradition I learned in the East it is the highest form of yoga, consisting of a body of secret doctrines, which are passed verbally from teacher to disciple. The avatara is one with a highly evolved soul and a pure, clean, virtually indestructible body[1] that is truly a temple for divinity. In my own definition, avatara yoga is a way of achieving the highest possible development of man, which includes mastery over passing time—that is, the ability to delay aging processes.

1. Some scientists think that the physical immortality of a man may be possible in the future.

Part One

Theory and Information

——

1

Physical Phenomena of Aging

With age even the most graceful, supple, and beautiful body changes its shape and becomes stiff. Its very texture changes. The smoothness and firmness of youth are gone, as if not only the skin but the flesh is different. In aging, the body goes through seven major changes:

1. Change in weight
2. Loss of suppleness
3. Change in texture (body firmness)
4. Loss of strength
5. Changes in the inner life of the body (circulation, respiration, digestion and elimination, reproduction [menopause and climacteric], metabolic processes)
6. Loss of energy
7. Decline of recuperative powers

Is it possible to delay these changes? Or even to arrest some of them completely? A careful study suggests a positive answer. For instance, the weight of the body, through diet, can be kept the same throughout one's adult lifetime. By regular exercises, suppleness in the joints can be retained. Although the body can't retain youthful firmness throughout its lifetime, flabbiness and loss of strength can be alleviated considerably by exercising various groups of muscles. Thus, two aspects of aging—the gaining of weight and the loss of suppleness—can be completely arrested by the normally healthy person. Flabbiness and loss of muscular strength can be delayed. That leaves us with the changes in the inner life of the body and loss of energy. To retain the efficiency of the bodily functions throughout life is the greatest challenge, yet yoga has an answer. Further, in many astonishing ways, the techniques of ancient yoga correspond to the most recent findings of modern science.

It is common knowledge in modern science that aging starts in the very cells of the body. As the youthful human body grows toward maturity, new cells outnumber dying cells. As one matures, a balance in the number of growing and dying cells is reached. In aging, the dying cells begin to outnumber those being born. For reasons yet unknown, cells stop duplicating themselves after a certain period, ultimately resulting in death.

The ancient world does not possess electronic microscopes and modern laboratories, yet everything in the study of yoga suggests the most profound knowledge of the functioning of the human body and the laws governing its growth, maturity, and aging. A number of yogic methods directly related to prolonging life and delaying aging correspond to modern ideas. For instance, some gerontologists recently suggested that if the temperature of the body could be lowered by one or two degrees, the life expectancy of mankind could be raised to 150 years. They do not know as yet how to do it. In yoga, breathing exercises for cooling the body, many hundreds of years old, suggest that the yogis knew the desirability of lowering body temperature to retard aging. Furthermore, they offer a method for doing it.

Modern science has discovered a factor related to rejuvenation and prolonging life in the medulla oblongata, commonly known as the "little brain." The medulla is believed to manufacture a "youth factor" hormone. With the passage of years the medulla gets progressively lazier in its production of this substance, thus accelerating the aging process. Scientific data suggest that aging could be delayed by mild electrical stimulation to the medulla. In yoga one of the poses for delaying aging is a certain inverted position of the body which stimulates the medulla, not by electricity (unknown to the ancients), but by extensive flow of arterial blood into that area.

Another corollary between modern science and yoga is the following: Scientists know that the brain cells are incapable of rejuvenation and that after a certain age they start to die at an astonishing rate. Some scientists think that this degeneration of the brain is the main factor in aging. Science has also taught us that the gray matter of the brain is completely dependent on oxygen. On the average the brain weighs only three pounds, yet it consumes between one-fourth and one-fifth of the oxygen used by the entire body. In the light of these scientific discoveries, the inverted poses of physical yoga, including the celebrated head pose known as the "king of all yoga postures," have acquired a new meaning. Apparently the ancients knew about the role of the brain in the aging process and the brain's dependency on oxygen, because quite a number of yoga techniques were designed to nourish the brain by creating an extra flow of well-oxygenated arterial blood to that organ. Recent experiments in the United States with elderly people who were developing senility syndromes involved their inhalation of pure oxygen, which arrested and even reversed, to some extent, the symptoms of senility.

Yet another similarity between modern science and ancient thought involves lowering the caloric level of

our diet as a means of delaying aging. Scientifically controlled experiments with the reduction of diet throughout
a lifetime have never been done with humans, yet most
dietitians agree that we overeat, digging our premature
graves with our knives and forks. Some dietitians suggest
that in affluent countries like America, people habitually
eat four times as much as they require. Scientists experimenting with animals discovered that the age of mice
could be doubled by reducing the diet to slightly more
than a starvation level. This method corresponds to the
first and main dogma of the yogic diet, which follows
the teaching that one should never overeat.

Now that we have seen some of the ways in which
modern science has furnished data to support certain
practices related to rejuvenation and retarding aging that
can be found in schools of yoga, let's have a closer look
at the changes in the human body that are associated
with aging.

Change in Weight

As the years pass, people usually become heavier. A European statistical report indicated that some 83 percent
of the population increase their weight, while the remaining 17 percent either become thinner or remain the
same. Increase in size as one ages occurs not vertically
but horizontally. Faces become broader and beefier, double chins appear, and the face seems to grow generally
less spiritual looking. Often ears and noses increase in
size, losing their once-graceful contours. Shoulders become thicker, the chest soft and flabby; the waist disap-
pears and is replaced by voluminous pouches full of fat
and gases. Legs affected by weight seem shorter. Fallen
arches and varicose veins appear as age advances.

Increased body weight leads to many other harmful
disorders: Fat people often have difficulty in breathing;

their hearts are affected, and their livers and kidneys become overstrained through regular overeating. The entire digestive system becomes clogged with impurities, resulting in a florid complexion and a bloated, unhealthy look. The skeletal structure is adversely affected by additional pressure on the spine as it supports the extra weight. Many cases of severe and otherwise unexplainable backaches are traced to this fact. In cases of gross obesity the weakened abdominal muscles which normally act as a "supporting belt" for the vital organs of the abdomen cannot perform their task efficiently. The bowels and stomach become pronouncedly displaced outside the normal body framework, resulting in serious and painful maladies.

Apart from rare instances of glandular disorders, weight is easy to control; to retain the same weight during a lifetime is a fairly simple matter. Avatara yoga teaches that upon reaching physical maturity, the body weight should remain the same throughout the rest of one's lifetime. Modern dietitians completely agree with this idea, suggesting that even a few pounds over the normal weight affects the physical condition unfavorably. Apart from checking weight regularly, a "pinch test" is recommended for correct evaluation of body weight. In this test, one stands in an upright position and pinches the skin in the region of the navel. If the fold is more than half an inch thick, it indicates an accumulation of extra fat. Increase in weight is a serious but unnecessary problem, as we shall see.

Loss of Suppleness

Another manifestation of aging is the progressive stiffening of the joints in the body, particularly in the spinal cord. This stiffening starts fairly early in life, becoming quite pronounced in most people by the age of forty.

Then, if nothing is done to arrest the process, it becomes more pronounced, leading to many other disorders caused by loss of body mobility. Occasionally joints deteriorate, welding together and creating painful inflammations that require prolonged treatments and even hospitalization. Arthritis and rheumatism are among the most painful and most widespread diseases of older people; in a great number of cases these could be prevented by systematic exercising of the joints. Stiffening of the body is accepted as inevitable by most people, who do not realize that this process can not only be brought to a standstill but actually reversed.

An ancient yogic proverb says, "A healthy spine is a healthy body." Many old as well as new schools of thought suggest manipulation or massage of the spine as a means of restoring the body to health. A stiff spine affects the whole inner life of the body, and in many instances the entire sympathetic nervous system becomes affected. Many techniques in yoga are centered around the spinal column, stretching and twisting it in order to maintain its flexibility. Stiffening of the spinal column has a direct connection with aging, and in that context "old age" comes with a stiff backbone. A youthful body is a supple body, and by preventing rigidity, old age can be kept successfully at bay. Nine out of ten people can regain suppleness by wise dieting and exercising.

Change in Texture (Body Firmness)

The most visible and distressing sign of aging is change in the bodily texture. Once firm and smooth, the body begins to lose its firmness sometimes in the early twenties. Lack of exercise causes deterioration of the muscles, which, in turn, affects the condition of the skin, causing a flabby, loose bodily appearance. The facial muscles also lose firmness, and the gravitational pull is plainly visible in a drawn and sagging look. Practically every part of the body loses its textural firmness, but the loss is most apparent on the inside of the upper arms, in the chest, stomach, buttocks, and the inner parts of the thighs. Directly and indirectly, weakening of the muscles causes the joints to fall out of alignment.

Hundreds of years before modern bodily and facial isometrics were introduced, Taoist yogis knew how to "sculpt" the body and they possessed a set of facial exercises to retain firmness. Changes in the texture of the body can never be stopped completely, but they can be delayed for a considerable time, resulting for the mature man in the beautiful look of Michelangelo's *Moses* and in the woman the look of a mature but still beautiful Aphrodite.

Loss of Strength

Deterioration of the muscles has a direct relation to the strength of the body. Even if the body weight is the same, the beautiful sensation of buoyancy and lightness is gone, as if the gravitational pull has increased twofold. Focusing on it as a major adverse change in the body, yogis have devised many techniques to maintain the wonderful sensation of lightness throughout a lifetime. Relative bodily strength (relationship between the muscles and the weight of the body) is maintained by practicing "raised *asanas,*" most of them with names of birds, suggesting the idea of lightness. Cycles of exercises not unlike modern isometrics are methodically practiced, along with various mental techniques to support the physical work.

Changes in the Inner Life of the Body

The "inner life of the body" includes circulation, respiration, digestion and elimination, reproduction, recuperative powers, and metabolic processes. Every one of these functions is affected by the passage of time. Circulation becomes sluggish, breathing becomes more and more shallow, digestion and elimination become problematical, sexual and recuperative powers diminish, and metabolism becomes pronouncedly slower, resulting, in many cases, in the accumulation of weight. Looking in more detail at the effects of aging on the inner life of the body, I will indicate briefly in each case how yogic techniques have evolved to cope with these difficulties.

Circulation

Poor circulation accounts for many syndromes of aging, such as cold in the extremities of the body and the development of varicose veins. Poor nourishment of the body cells causes the skin to become dry and develop wrinkles. An inadequate supply of rich arterial blood to the roots of the spinal nerves adversely affects the entire sympathetic nervous system. Bad circulation also causes the endocrine glands to malfunction. "We are as young as our glands," said Professor Serge Voronoff, one of the first gerontologists of the century, who suggested transplanting monkey glands into humans. Although he was the subject of ridicule and his methods never proved effective, many modern gerontologists agree that at least one of the secrets of human aging is to be found in the deterioration of the glands as a result of poor circulation.

Respiration

Respiration is badly affected in aging. People simply lose their ability to breathe deeply as their lives become more and more sedentary. They are no longer engaged in vigorous sports or physical activities. Their very mode of life precludes deep breathing, thus starting a vicious cycle: With shallow breathing, the bloodstream is not properly oxygenated or purified; the chemistry of the body is affected and, in turn, energy declines. The brain, denied an inadequate supply of oxygen, starts to deteriorate. Speech is impaired, as well as the sense of balance and orientation. Eyesight and hearing also deteriorate. Shallow breathing affects the posture. The rib cage shrinks, the chest becomes hollow, the back bent, the shoulders raised and immobile. Respiration has a direct connection with the cardiovascular system and, very often, the functioning of the heart is adversely affected by poor respiration.

In yoga, inadequate depth of breath is considered a typical manifestation of aging. Metaphysical teachings regarding respiration suggest that *shallow breathing is the root of all evil.* Yoga teaches that apart from the oxygenation of the bloodstream in breathing, we are also absorbing into our systems the universal energy, or life force, that is called *prana* in India and *chi* in China. Without regular deep breathing, the amount of life force in the human system diminishes, triggering in turn a movement toward senility. Ancient schools of thought are emphatic in teaching that the body can be rejuvenated by breathing exercises.

Digestion and Elimination

A cynical French anecdote says that joy in human life is threefold: In youth man finds most joy in good sex; in maturity he finds it in good food; in old age he finds it in good elimination. The anecdote accurately suggests the importance to the elderly of the process of elimination. In declining years, poor digestion is always connected with inadequate elimination. The inner cleanliness of the body is lost; the system becomes clogged with all kinds of impurities. Constipation, apart from its harm to the body, can be a source of misery to the mind as well. Constipation is a primary cause of hemorrhoids and, according to the naturopathic school, it affects the prostate gland. When digestion is faulty, one's whole digestive system and metabolism are thrown out of balance.

In the yogic tradition digestion is one of the energies of the body, referred to as *samana,* while the process of evicting waste matter is known as *apana. Samana-prana-apana* balance is one of the major principles in delaying aging. This subject will be dealt with at length in chapter 5 on rejuvenation.

Reproduction (Menopause and Climacteric)

In women, the time when menstruation ceases, thus terminating the childbearing period, occurs usually during the mid-forties. In most cases it is accompanied by physiological and psychological symptoms of distress: hot flashes, loss of energy, palpitations, giddiness, and, in some cases, insomnia. The psychological aspects of menopause often include irritability, tension, failing memory, and depression. The symptoms vary from woman to woman. Some women suffer very badly when passing through this change of life. Cases of mental illness are not unusual, though only a small percent result in analytical treatment.

Women who can adapt to new interests after their childbearing years suffer less than those who cannot. The introduction of hormone injections has greatly assisted women in overcoming the harmful effects of menopause, and yoga exercises can in many cases produce even more beneficial results. The psychological effects of menopause can be corrected successfully by regular practice of certain mental exercises that help one to achieve a more positive and philosophical attitude toward living.

In men the climacteric occurs later than menopause in women, usually in the late fifties or sixties. It involves a loss of sexual drive, semi-impotence, a sensation of tiredness, and loss of sleep. In many cases the prostate gland becomes a problem. It increases in size, either causing difficulty in passing water or causing irritation of the bladder, resulting in increased frequency of urination. The psychological manifestations of aging often are even more pronounced in men than in women. A man tends to brood, become gloomy, bored, or irritable. He often feels that he is a failure, that his life is over, and his ego feels dangerously threatened. On occasion this syndrome even leads to suicide. Yoga exercises stimulating the endocrine glands give one ideal antidote to the climacteric.

Another aspect of aging is the imbalance of male-female hormones in the human system. We know that the most "feminine" woman has some masculine qualities, and even the most "masculine" male has some feminine characteristics. With the passage of years a person's contrasexual qualities emerge more strongly. Masculine characteristics diminish in men and more feminine ones emerge; conversely, feminine qualities diminish in women and masculine traits appear. I have seen fearless British colonels retired from Indian service taking to embroidery and knitting and bursting into tears at the slightest provocation, while many once lovely women start to grow facial hair and their once gentle voices become hoarse and abrasive.

Taoist yoga offers the yin-yang pose to prevent these changes, suggesting that this aspect of aging was well known by the sages of Taoist yoga. Tantra yoga (liberation of the spirit by sexual union) has an especially wide range of techniques for accumulating sexual energy and is capable of literally reversing the decline of sexual power.

Through these practices the female can prolong her procreative period and painlessly make the transition to the postchildbearing years. As with the male, the joy of sex can be available practically throughout her entire lifetime.

Metabolic Processes

Generally speaking, with advancing years the body becomes less efficient at converting food into energy and in preparing it to be stored for later use. People eat more than they require, thus creating the wrong balance between intake and output of energy. There is at least one theory that aging can be traced to the failure of the body to rid itself of accumulated metabolic products. When the body is strained by any kind of excess, whether work, pleasure, or pain, its metabolic rate goes up and produces more oxidation products than it can eliminate efficiently. The antidote, of course, is rest, especially after vigorous activity. One must give the body time to metabolize at its own pace. It has also been suggested that metabolism works better in cool surroundings and that a lower body temperature greatly aids the process.

The curative power of rest and sleep is important to yogic teachings, and the lowering of body temperature is a feature of some yogic practices. Yoga also teaches many ways of purifying the body of waste. Thus the exercises offer many ways of improving metabolism.

Loss of Energy

Most of the symptoms of aging we have looked at so far can be traced directly to a falling off of energy during the passing of years. If you want to see energy in motion, look at a child: His little body explodes in movement like fireworks going off. Contrast that with the sedentary middle-aged businessman or the doddering old person confined to a nursing home because he can no longer take care of himself. We think of an inactive child as a sickly child, but we accept relative inactivity in adulthood as inevitable.

Loss of energy prevents one from the regular, vigorous movement necessary to good metabolism, steady weight, and supple muscles. I believe that faulty breathing habits are the main cause of loss of energy. People in the West know next to nothing about breathing properly. In the East, breathing is the highest physical, mental, and spiritual discipline. Westerners who can learn to breathe properly can live a more energetic life. By keeping one's energy level high, one can exercise to keep good muscle tone as well as bodily strength and firm texture. Energetic movement causes one to burn calories and thus control weight. Better oxygenation of the blood furnishes the inner organs and nerve cells with richer nourishment, thus enabling them to function more efficiently and to create even more energy. The vicious cycle of losing energy can be turned around to gaining energy through proper breathing.

Decline of Recuperative Powers

Another sign of aging is the decline of the body's recuperative powers. In elderly people, injuries to the skin will not heal as readily as in youth, while bruising of the body becomes much easier and more painful. Older people succumb to infectious diseases more readily than young people, and they shake them off with much greater difficulty. Although young people, even children, can fall victim to cancer, it is basically a disease of old age. Among older people, even if a disease is finally overcome, it leaves the person weaker, as if complete recuperation were not possible. This all points to the loss of basic energy in the human system and will be discussed in Chapter 5 on healing.

The psychological determination needed for recuperation is often in short supply during one's later years, when a good deal of the joy of living is lost. The unconscious and conscious willingness to participate in the adventure of life declines. According to the Greek philosopher Plutarch, the right time to die is when you don't want to live anymore. By having our bodies in much better condition, the frontiers of old age can be pushed back, extending our desire to live fully well into the period now associated with senility.

Summary

Studying the physical phenomena of aging, we could come to the conclusion that all these aspects of aging shouldn't be taken as inevitable, but that they could be delayed and even reversed by gaining a better knowledge of the body's needs and functioning and by learning and practicing techniques for meeting these needs more efficiently. In the entire animal world, man is the only species who can challenge Father Time. Instead of meekly succumbing to conventional and, in my opinion, absurd notions of aging, man can win for himself many more years for mental and spiritual development by taking better care of his body.

The body and mind are intricately interrelated. Staying young mentally is a medically acknowledged factor of staying young physically. Many doctors today teach that we shouldn't give up youth so readily. Inquisitiveness and alertness of spirit should have no cutoff point in age. That is the subject of the next chapter.

2

Psychological Phenomena
of Aging

The aging process includes loss of certain mental faculties such as failing memory, poor concentration, inflexible habits of thought, and the inability sometimes even to comprehend innovative thought or behavior. Most of these aging syndromes are inevitably associated with senility, but they often begin long before a person becomes technically senile.

Old age has a strange effect on the memory. Many elderly people literally cannot recall what they were doing yesterday and at the same time are besieged with vivid memories of events that occurred forty or fifty years ago. The "retrospective memory" that emerges removes the person from present or future considerations as he becomes engrossed in the past. Many elderly people live these early memories again and again, brooding over their mistakes, powerless now to make changes, and depressed by their helplessness. This syndrome of aging is described with great poignance by Ingmar Bergman in his classic film *Wild Strawberries,* in which bittersweet memories flood into the elderly man's mind as he moves across the European landscape.

While we are young we are able to push into the unconscious all those items that we do not wish to recall. But with age, these repressed contents usurp the ego's control and present themselves to consciousness in all their unpleasantness: memories of offenses we have committed, emotional pains we have suffered, and perhaps worst of all, moments when we have failed to be all that we could have been in love or work or play. The nineteenth-century Russian poet A. Apuchtin expresses the old man's dilemma:

> Black thoughts, like swarms of merciless flies,
> Do not let me sleep all night.
> Around my head they circle and sting.
> The moment I chase one away
> I am stabbed in the heart by another.
> Their continuous passing
> Brings me closer and closer to the abyss of despair.

Such memories demand attention. Unable to assuage them, old people spend many nights wracked with insomnia.

For an old person, living in the past becomes more regular as the ability to concentrate weakens. He drifts away from the present challenge to change and grow. The natural drive to expand the youthful inquiring mind has been replaced by a stubborn unwillingness to admit any idea that comes from outside one's already acquired knowledge. This condition is described humorously in an Oriental proverb: "The old ass wouldn't move even if whacked with a pole."

Besides poor memory and concentration, old people often develop a tendency toward miserliness and toward a set of worries and fears that is virtually intolerable to them and incomprehensible to those around them. The universality of these fears is demonstrated by the yogic tradition, which admonishes a man to guard against these fears in old age: the fear of losing possessions, the fear of losing health, the fear of loneliness, the fear of aging, and the fear of death. Many factors are responsible for the negative aspects of aging. One's state of mind is crucial. We can look happily toward maturity only if we have a philosophy to carry us forward.

With the passage of years a certain reassessment of values occurs. Man's ego development is on the decline; he is not interested in engaging in strenuous battles to establish himself as a businessman, a politician, or a lover. His eyes are opening inwardly, and through the development of inner vision his mental horizons are broadened and his spiritual development advances. His physical eyes may not be as good as in younger years but, with the new inner vision acquired, the entire world looks more meaningful. This is the beginning of the birth of the spiritual man out of the physical man so eloquently described by St. Paul in his message to the Corinthians and by the sage Patangali in his aphorisms.

C. G. Jung, the eminent Swiss psychiatrist, corroborates these observations regarding midlife changes as they occur in both men and women. Jung asserts:

For a young person it is almost a sin, or at least a danger, to be too preoccupied with himself; but for the aging person it is a duty and a necessity to devote serious attention to himself. After having lavished its light upon the world, the sun withdraws its rays in order to illuminate itself. Instead of doing likewise, many old people prefer to be hypochondriacs, niggards, pedants, applauders of the past or else eternal adolescents—all lamentable substitutes for the illumination of the self, but inevitable consequences of the delusion that the second half of life must be governed by the principles of the first.[1]

1. C. G. Jung, *Collected Works,* vol. 8, *The Structure and Dynamics of the Psyche* (Princeton: Princeton University Press, 1969), p. 399.

Jung then makes an intriguing distinction between nature and culture and shows their relationship to aging in the individual. He says, "Money-making, social achievement, family and posterity are nothing but plain nature, not culture. Culture lies outside the purpose of nature. Could by any chance culture be the meaning and purpose of the second half of life?"[2]

Self-illumination through the pursuit of wisdom and culture is, in my opinion, the primary purpose of life during and beyond middle age. Yet, can one pursue this or any other goal if one is in poor health? On the contrary, poor health leads the aging person to the wrong kind of self-centeredness. We have all seen and heard old people who are preoccupied with their own physical symptoms, who will sit all day and talk about their aches and pains, about what is wrong with their digestion and their diet. This type of old person is a burden to everyone, including himself. Many young people observe this behavior and think they learn that this is what old age will inevitably be like. Small wonder that old age is so feared in America when young people have so many bad examples to teach them about the nature of aging.

Let us consider for a moment what old age might be like if it is seen from a positive viewpoint. Starting perhaps at age fifty, there might be a normal process of disengagement from the style of life one has established up to that point. The housewife might have finished her child rearing and sent her children out into the world on their own. She will feel a vacuum in her life, but at the same time she might well feel a certain sense of relief. Her husband might have established himself some years ago in his career and, if so, will be thinking about disengaging himself from burdens, perhaps those of his very success. Many of his financial obligations connected with the sup-

2. Ibid., p. 400.

port of his family will be fulfilled, and further money-making efforts may seem relatively purposeless now that his children are independent, his home is paid for, and so on. At this point in life men and women undergo a major crisis in their external environment as well as in their physical bodies. The "change of life" is a very great change indeed, and it furthers one to have a clear idea of what one is changing from and what sort of new goals are proper. I believe that the pursuit of cultural interests and the achievement of personal wisdom are the primary goals of the second half of life. But to pursue these goals, one must have a healthy body. The human body is literally what keeps us in this world, and the quality of one's life experiences is profoundly influenced throughout by the condition of one's physical self.

In a way, the yogic point of view could be compared to the classical Greek triangle where the base is the body, one side is the mind, and the other side is the spirit. If the base is destroyed prematurely, the mind never has a chance to complete its development, and the spirit is released far too early. The whole structure then lies in ruins.

Usually, people mellow with the passage of time, but not always. Quite often an ambitious, hard-driving businessman is transformed into a remorseless, angry old man full of hatred of youth and new ideas. This phenomenon is the other side of the coin of self-pity: He is still too strong to pity himself, but he knows he is on the decline and blames the whole world for it. On the other hand, a considerable number of old people like to be fussed over. Many mothers and fathers ruin the lives of their children by playing the same record ("I will die soon") all the time.

All that is quite unnecessary. Old age, in its own way, could be the best part of life, the culmination of a long journey full of serenity, wisdom, and spirituality. We have many examples of people growing old in such a way. Albert Schweitzer in his eighties was still working almost twenty hours a day. Leopold Stokowski was a dedicated master of his art in his nineties. Artur Rubinstein, Georgia O'Keeffe, and Eubie Blake are still examples to us of creative old people. Philosophers, scientists, artists—people generally dedicated to the creative aspects of life—often experience this longevity and excellent health.

When the richness and excitement of the second half of life can in some way be visualized by the individual, the challenge becomes one of physically enduring for the purpose of realizing mental and spiritual growth. Winning precious years from Father Time so that one can read more books, travel, attend lectures, cultivate latent talents in music, art, or science, follow up interests that were suppressed because of the needs of the first half of life—that is what aging means. If one's physical body is in good condition, then one's senses are keen instruments that willingly lend themselves to the journey toward wisdom. To meet the challenge of the second half of life, all of one's strength is required. And the wonderful paradox is that the more one's strength is used, the more it is retained. Those who shrink away from the goals of the second half of life destroy themselves through atrophy and negativity just as surely as those who shrink away from the goals of the first half of life. Those who embrace their goals dilate their energies through purposeful living. Naturally, those who live purposefully will be the very ones who will want to extend their lifetime. Observing themselves growing each day in knowledge and wisdom motivates them to extend the number of their days. Seen in this light, it is no wonder that the yogic disciplines of delaying aging originated and were perfected in the East, where spiritual growth has been seen as the end and aim of life for perhaps forty centuries.

Life is a great university that teaches us many remarkable things. In metaphysical traditions, it teaches us that physical expiration is but the beginning of a new experience on a higher plane unknown to the living. In many traditions of East and West, the second part of human life is preparation for death. Tibetan yoga teaches a famous *bordo* (the art of dying) which actually prepares people for a new life in the world beyond. Its main doctrine teaches that every one of us experiences two great events: birth—our appearance in this world—and death— our exit from it. All other events pale by comparison. In both cases, we need help. Mother, midwife, and doctor help the child enter the world. In the Christian tradition priests attend the dying. In Tibetan yoga trained lamas assist the dying person during his last hours before his exit from this life. If a man is prepared, this exit is painless, beautiful, and full of inner meaning. In the context of this book, this attitude toward death is important in contributing to serenity and longevity.

I have presented in this chapter what I believe to be the most important aspects of the mental phenomena of aging, both the failure of certain mental faculties and the inadequacy of personal philosophy, in many cases, to carry us forward with a sense of expectation and promise of the riches of mature life. However, it is possible to transform both our attitudes toward old age and the condition of our bodies, thereby prolonging and enriching the years of our maturity.

Part Two

How to Reverse
the Biological Clock

3

Reprogramming Oneself About Age

As was briefly mentioned in the Preface, the secret of slowing down the aging process is a clear understanding of the difference between the chronological and the biological ages of the body. There are "young" old people and "old" young people. One of my teachers in China was a man reputed to be 110 years of age, yet his biological age was perhaps 60. He was supple, agile, energetic, strong, and possessed unusual stamina. He had good eyesight, hearing, and unusually youthful skin. If he were to be examined by a Western gerontologist, his age most likely would be seen as fifty years younger than his actual chronological age.

In avatara yoga the student is trained to forget how old he is in years. He is taught to think of himself in strictly biological terms. His entire psyche is reprogrammed. By detaching himself from his chronological age, he causes a number of remarkable changes to take place. Let's examine this phenomenon more closely.

The average life span in the United States for a man is seventy-one years. Imagine a man of sixty-nine who is all the time conscious that he *is* sixty-nine. He knows that on the average he will have only two years to live.

If he surpasses the age of seventy-one, he will thereafter be conscious that he is living on borrowed time. Consciously and unconsciously, he remains close to the idea of death. That situation exists for every senior citizen, and very often consciousness of the chronological age plays havoc with the lives of younger people as well. How often we hear from a man of forty, "I am too old to play tennis. It's too strenuous. I'd better switch to golf." Throughout his lifetime, a man is hypnotized by the figure of his chronological age. For women, the mark of forty is a crucial rubicon full of unhappiness and menace. Women in their thirties envy women in their twenties, and some women in their twenties envy girls in their teens. We would be much happier and healthier if we could reprogram ourselves regarding chronological and biological ages.

In Western culture we can discern among mature people typical patterns of behavior that carry them too rapidly into old age. One simple but vivid example is the tendency of people past fifty suddenly to begin dressing like "old folks." Women become more and more conservative, choosing colorless and poorly designed clothes in order not to attract attention to themselves. Men, on the other hand, often adorn themselves in clownish outfits— bold colors and large checks or stripes—as if their age carried the privilege of looking absurd. In either case, our mode of dress is a way of identifying with an age group. We need to be aware of falling into the pattern of saying, "I'm too old to wear that," or "I can get away with looking clownish because I'm past the age when anybody cares." Of course, we don't want to go to the foolish extreme of imitating teenagers, but there is no real reason why all adults shouldn't choose from the same fashions those that suit each personality best, regardless of age. How refreshing it is to encounter a mature man or woman who has retained a sense of style in dress! Older people who have kept themselves trim and supple can be immensely attractive, especially when they have the advantages over youth of experience, knowledge, and wit.

I am absolutely convinced that to think and to behave "old" will contribute to physical aging, while youthful behavior and identification with a younger generation can slow down the aging process. In that sense, the word *neoteny*, which is usually used to refer to the carrying over of some larval or immature characteristics into the adult stage, acquires a positive rather than a negative meaning. This word was used by anthropologist Ashley Montagu to describe the process of retaining youthful characteristics as late as possible into adult life. Many modern psychiatrists agree that the mental rigidity acquired in the passage of years is quite detrimental to mental and physical health.

The retention of childlike qualities in the psyche was seen by Chinese philosophers as the most important part of spiritual growth: to keep an open mind throughout the journey of life; to retain the inability to lie, to cheat, to harm others or ourselves. These are qualities to be cultivated rather than lost.

The way we dress is only one example of our tendency to rush into old age. There are other subtle ways in which we begin to age too rapidly. Some habits that contribute to this syndrome begin in youth, when we sometimes seek to appear more mature than we are in order to acquire greater social ease. For instance, I believe that when a young man puts a pipe into his mouth for the first time, at that instant he becomes ten years older. Unconsciously, something happens to his psyche. He identifies himself with a "wise old man," serene, contemplating the problems of life while comfortably nestled in an armchair and rhythmically puffing away.

I remember very well one of the boys with whom I graduated from high school in China. He was an intelligent and gifted young man, among the first ten in my class. But there was something peculiar in his behavior: He seemed constantly to be portraying a much older person. It has since occurred to me that he might have been experiencing this premature aging because of excessive identification with his father, who was even then an elderly man, or with his grandfather, whom he also imitated. I ran into my former classmate several times over a period of perhaps thirty years. Each time I was struck with how quickly he had "aged." At forty-five he looked like a man of sixty. I could not believe that at one time we shared the same desk. He died at age fifty-two from multiple causes, problems usually associated with old age (coronary insufficiency and high blood pressure, for example). I am certain that his premature death came from the pattern of behavior he adopted from his father when he was much too young to behave that way. He lost his youth without ever having experienced it.

Just as we can acquire habits that cause us to age too quickly, we can break habits and regain a certain amount of youth. I remember visiting one of my friends, a lawyer, who at that time was about sixty. He greeted me in an unusually happy frame of mind and said, "Do you know, I am feeling thirty years younger today." When I inquired what was behind his youthful exuberance he told me simply, "For the first time in my life, I put on a pair of jeans." Some impulse had caused him to step into his son's jeans. They fit him perfectly. He felt a remarkable transformation and a recovery of years in his life.

Imagine a person born on an uninhabited island surviving into his manhood and maturity: With no knowledge of his date of birth and projected time of death in the future, he would be much closer to the idea of immortality than we are. Our dates of birth, our concept of years, months, hours, are sinister reminders of our mortality because most people remain conscious all the time of how old they are. I was trained to think of myself in terms of biological age only—to measure my age only in terms of my condition and well-being. Today, in my senior years, I never feel older than when I was in my twenties.

Philosophically, there is something within us that never ages. The spirit is immortal and indestructible, according to many religious beliefs; it can't get old. We can train ourselves to think young, and the entire tone of our physical and psychological well-being will improve.

Chronological and Biological Age

Looking somewhat closer, we could conclude that man has not two, but three different ages: chronological, biological, and mental (not in the context of advanced or retarded intellect, but in terms of his *joie de vivre*). Turning back the biological clock must start in the psyche, by identifying your true age as the condition of your body. When this is done, all you have to do is to learn methods for improving your condition, day after day rebuilding your body. Willpower, perseverance, and belief in the ultimate success of your program could become the most fascinating game you ever played in your life, especially when you become conscious that the biological clock really is moving backward. The sensing of possible victory is a great inspiration.

We are all passing through the stages of youth, maturity, and old age. You can prolong youth if you start young; you can prolong the productive part of your life if you start at maturity; and you can actually grow younger if you start late in life. This contest with Father Time is equally enjoyable for people in all age groups.

Many scientists today agree that, removing self-imposed obstacles, the normal span of a man's life is between 120 and 130 years. There are today in three areas of the world (the Caucasus in Russia, the Himalayas in India, and the Andes in South America) "pockets" of people whose average life span far surpasses our own. In their populations, the number of people over 100 is remarkable. This confirms that our life expectancy is unnaturally short. How are these villagers different from us? Let me give just one example. People in these mountainous areas from early childhood walk steep paths inhaling pure mountain air, which purifies the cells of their bodies and gives them large amounts of energy to live on. If, as I have suggested, the main cause of aging is faulty and inadequate breathing, we can see how these people have at least one advantage over us.

The Importance of Attitudes

We are all aging prematurely, and we should realize that this is an unnatural phenomenon that could be corrected through appropriate knowledge. Some gerontologists go so far as to give actual figures concerning how normal age is shortened ten to fifteen years by smoking, ten years by excessive drinking, ten to fifteen years by overeating, and ten to fifteen years by breathing polluted air. If you add all these years to the so-called normal span of seventy-one, you will come close to the yogic calculations of the potentially normal life span.

A cat's body grows about one year, and it lives an average of ten; a dog grows a year and lives perhaps thirteen. If we take this ratio of one year of growth to ten years of life, imagine the potential of man's life span when we consider that he spends twenty-five years growing!

In yogic thought the life span is given as about 150 years. Lately, many scientists are inclined to accept that as something feasible in the not-so-distant future. At the turn of the century the average life span in the United States was forty-five. Today it is over seventy. It is only logical to assume that in several generations it will be over 100. With that change, most of our modern ideas of aging will be dissolved. Today we think we are young in our twenties, middle-aged in our forties, and old in our sixties. With the life span extended to over 100, youth could be prolonged into the forties, middle years well into the sixties, and old age would begin in the eighties or nineties. Still further in time, it could be a very different world—a world of beautiful women and handsome men in their seventies, with Wimbledon tennis and Olympic games played by athletes in their sixties.

Perhaps the most fascinating theoretical finding of modern research regarding aging teaches that aging is accelerated by numerous causes and that prevention of only 10 percent of all causes of aging could lead to an average life span of about 170 years. This statement leads to the logical conclusion that if elimination of 10 percent of the causes of old age could increase the life span by 100 years, the elimination of 90 percent could increase it by 900 years. This prospect startles into my mind a teaching that rings throughout avatara yoga: that the age of a highly evolved human could be extended into hundreds of years and, potentially, one could become immortal. Legends of India, Tibet, and China are full of references to famous sages up to 700 years old. Again, science confirms at least the theoretical possibility of such a fantastic expansion of longevity.

All this speculation is about the future, of course. My main point in this book is that disciplines of three yogas (Indian, Chinese, Tibetan) offer much information about how the biological clock can be reversed *now*. In my experience as a teacher of yoga, I have seen many cases of people turning back the biological clock. Any serious and dedicated student can achieve success in direct proportion to the physical and mental effort put into his study.

4

The Breath of Life

The breath of life moves through a deathless valley
Of eternal motherhood
Which conceives and bears the seed of life.
The seeming of a world never to stop,
For men to draw breath as they will:
The more they take of it, the more remains.

—Lao-tzu

From the first inhalation of the newly born child to the last expiration of a dying man, breath is synonymous with life. That is why in the yogic tradition the life span is expressed not by *years* but by *number of breaths.* Considering that life cannot exist without breath, it will very likely puzzle future historians that we in the West are almost completely ignorant not only of how to breathe correctly but even of the mechanics of breathing. Many instances have been recorded wherein men have survived without food for forty days. By contrast, we cannot survive without air for five minutes, and yet we don't know how to breathe correctly. Apart from some biology textbooks containing studies of the respiratory system, very few books on breathing have been written.

In the West some recognition of the curative effect of breathing fresh mountain air has been made in such places as tuberculosis sanitoriums. Still, the enormous potential for health and rejuvenation through breath control remains largely unexplored in the West. In the East, however, there is a tradition of many centuries of acquired knowledge about breathing. The ancient Egyptians sought the secret of life in breathing, as did the Chinese, Indian, and Tibetan sages. Ancient yoga treatises on breathing are written in metaphysical terms to protect accumulated knowledge from misuse by the ignorant.

Hathayoga Pradipika, one of the classical treatises, voices a strong warning:

As the lion, elephant and tiger can become tame only very gradually, so also must be treated the *vaya* [vital air]: otherwise it kills the practicer.

Decoding this warning suggests the enormous power of breath controls and its grave dangers if they are done incorrectly.[1]

The Relationship Between Breath and Life

In discussing various breath controls, physiology and the metaphysics of breathing have to be taken into consideration. Behind *all* breath controls is a profound knowledge of physiology, which is intricately interlaced with metaphysical teachings. In my opinion, what we term "metaphysics" today will become a part of scientific heritage tomorrow. The West needs to find a bridge to this ancient knowledge for the sake of its own scientific growth.

To provide a context for the exercises that follow, the

1. In the introduction to the chapter on advanced breath controls, I mention that I checked and rechecked my decoding of the ancient texts with the masters of three yogas and, only after being completely satisfied, present various exercises suitable for Western students.

main aspects of metaphysical teachings must be explained.[2]

Pranic Theory

Pranic theory is the cornerstone of these teachings. Sages of the past believed that in the air we breathe dwells a cosmic energy called *prana* in India, *chi* in China, and *ka* in Egypt. By improving the volume of our breathing, we could increase intake of this energy into our system, which breath by breath is stored in the solar plexus, or *Manipura* chakra in Indian tradition. It is also believed that by an appropriate effort of concentration this energy could be directed to any part of the body—vital organs, nerve centers, the very cells of the body—with energizing and invigorating effects.

Raja yoga, yoga of mental and spiritual development, teaches that we can develop our mental powers by breath; Kundalini yoga speaks of the latent possibilities of a man awakened by breath controls, while physical yoga believes that radiant health and longevity can be achieved by the same means.

Yoga teachings describe two important nerve channels, *ida* and *pingala,* that begin in our nostrils, branching into the upper cortex of the brain, then traveling down the spinal column, crisscrossing several times to form chakras, or centers of energy, and ultimately reaching the anus. These *nadis,* or nerve channels, make direct contact with the life force in the air as we breathe. If oxygen in the air purifies our bloodstream, *prana* energizes the entire nervous system of the body.[3]

2. The yogic concept of human nature would require volumes to explicate meaningfully, and I don't intend to get deep into the subject here.
3. The English terms "cosmic energy" and "life force" have no importance in our culture equivalent to the importance of *prana* and *chi* in Oriental cultures. Since the Indian word is more familiarly used in discussions of yoga to designate energy or life force in the air, I will use *prana* in my subsequent references to this essential principle of yogic practices.

Pingala (in the right nostril) is symbolically linked to masculine forces both abstract and specific, both to maleness and to masculine aspects of heat, strength, and energy, whereas *ida* (in the left nostril) is linked to femaleness and to the feminine aspects of coolness, gentleness, and compassion. Unification of breaths through these two channels is a fundamental principle of yoga, which, in fact, means unity.[4] The inner structure of man is an interplay of the forces represented by these two nerves located in our nostrils.[5]

Chakras

The chakras,[6] psychic centers of the body, play a very important part in higher breathing practices. They react to intensive flow of *prana*, directed by concentration of thought. To a certain extent they correspond to the nervous centers of the physical body.

Literally, the word *chakra* means a "wheel," a center of energy, and according to esoteric belief, they are organs of the second, or ethereal, body of a man.

There are seven main chakras set one above the other (fig. 1), each drawn in the form of a lotus with a different number of petals, containing a different number of Sanskrit letters or characters in its center. Each of these centers has a different color. Going from the base of the spine up, they are *Muladara* (root center), located between anus and genitals, called the *yoni* place in India. Metaphysically it is the seat of Kundalini, power symbol-

4. The right nostril is a "sun" nostril, *ha* in Sanskrit, while the left one is a "moon" nostril, *tha* in Sanskrit. Hatha yoga or physical yoga is unification of breath through the right and left nostrils.

5. Mercury's wand, which many pharmacies have as their insignia, may in fact be a picture of the spinal cord, with the two main nerves of the sympathetic nervous system crisscrossing.

6. The physical aspects are described on pages 99–102 on advanced breathing exercises.

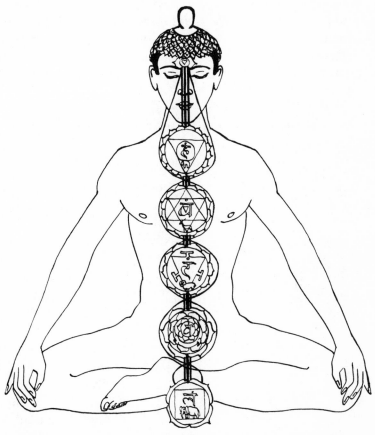

Chakras or psychic nervous centers in metaphysical anatomy. (*Drawing by Daphne Hewson*)

ized as a sleeping serpent coiled three and a half times around the base of the spine. Vibration of energy in this chakra is low, and on the physical plane it is the seat of *apana* (excretory power) and associated with inner cleanliness of the body.

The next chakra, *Svadisthana* (support of life breath), is located in the genitals and associated with erotic desire.

The *Manipura* (lotus of the navel) is located in the solar plexus. It is the seat of physical energy in the body, driving power, energy of the ego.

These lower chakras are activated by desires of "worldly" pursuits—food, comfort, sex, social powers. They are practically devoid of spiritual qualities, and it is taught that spiritually undeveloped people have only these chakras vibrating.

The *Anahata* chakra (unstruck sound) corresponds with the cardiac plexus. This is a higher chakra and its vibrations are more refined. Activation of this chakra is the beginning of spiritual awakening.

Vishuddha chakra (center of great purity) is located in the region of the thyroid gland. It is known as the gate to spiritual enlightenment, and the vibrations of this center are even more refined.

Ajna chakra (center of command) is located between the eyebrows, and in mystical teachings it is referred to as the "third eye." It is a belief that this center corresponds with the pineal gland in the brain, according to some schools of thought, the dormant organ of higher faculties. Mystical tradition describes this center as a place of divine revelations and mystical ecstasy.

The seventh and most important center is the *Brahma* chakra (thousand-petaled lotus) in the upper cortex of the brain. Activation of this chakra completes the growth of spiritual man out of the physical and signifies full mental development.

Comparing the Indian tradition of activating chakras by breath controls with the Chinese school of thought, I found on many occasions that the basic principles are remarkably similar. In exercises of healing breaths *(chigoon)* certain centers in the body are stimulated by the energy of breath in very much the same way as they are stimulated in acupuncture. In these breathing exercises the acupuncturist's needle is replaced by the even sharper "needle" of mental concentration. A "beam" of cosmic energy, or *prana,* is directed with exhalation to these centers, energizing them and restoring healthy balance of the body.

Significantly, the art of healing breath is being restored in modern China. At present not less than thirty breathing clinics are in operation where people are treated for multitudes of maladies by breathing exercises, diet, and rest.

Physiology of Breathing

After outlining the main metaphysical ideas behind breathing practices, I would like to review the physiology of breathing as it is known to Western science. A basic knowledge of the subject will help the student to derive full benefit from the practices.

The "respiratory system" is a familiar term to everyone in the West who claims even a little formal education, yet we are constantly amazed at how confused our knowledge of the body becomes as we get away from the biology classroom. In my years of teaching yoga, having among my students people from many backgrounds, including doctors and scientists, I have never heard a correct description of breathing. People are vague even about such questions as whether we should inhale through the nose and exhale through the mouth, or vice versa. The very mechanics of inhalation and exhalation are either misunderstood or unknown by most people. To derive the full benefit from various breath control practices, the physiology of breathing must be clearly understood. The following is a simple description of how the respiratory system works.

First, we must remember that the human body is constructed of trillions of cells. In order to live, each cell must be fed oxygen and each cell must have the waste material it generates removed. These two needs are satisfied directly by our circulating bloodstream. Bright, richly oxygenated blood is pumped out of the heart through a system of arterial pathways to each individual cell. As the blood reaches each cell, it serves the dual function of feeding oxygen to the cell and removing the carbon dioxide waste. Becoming progressively laden with waste and reduced in oxygen content, the blood gradually loses its bright color. When the oxygen–carbon dioxide content reaches a certain balance, the blood is returned to the heart through a system of veins. The heart is a pump, however, and not an organ that serves directly to oxygenate and purify the blood. That crucial function is left to the lungs.

Air from the outside world is brought to the lungs through passageways linked together in the following order: first the nostrils, then the nasal passages, then the pharynx, the larynx, the trachea, and the bronchi. The passageways to the lungs serve a dual purpose: They warm the air before it reaches the lungs, and they remove some of the dust particles and bacteria that the air contains. Some of the dust particles and bacteria are prevented from reaching the lungs simply because the passageways are intricately twisted; others are trapped either by mucus or by cilia, tiny hairs that beat in a direction opposite to the incoming air. Oxygen is not taken from the air until the air reaches the air sacs, or alveoli, located in the lungs themselves. For oxygen to be taken from the outside air and brought into our bloodstream, a process of absorption is utilized. It has been estimated that the amount of surface area required to absorb the oxygen needed for all the body's trillions of cells would be about thirty times the surface area of the entire skin. This surface is furnished by the alveoli, which are amazingly thin and are folded compactly over and over upon themselves. The surface area covered by the membrane of the alveolar cells totals some 600 square feet.

When the air we breathe reaches the air sacs, a film of moisture covering the air sacs dissolves the oxygen. Minute blood vessels called capillaries are adjacent to the air sacs. Thus, two unbelievably thin membranes—those of the capillaries and those of the air sacs—are in direct contact. At the same moment that carbon dioxide is passed through the capillary walls into the air sacs, the dissolved oxygen is passed through the air sacs and then through the capillary walls into the bloodstream, where it is immediately absorbed by the blood's hemoglobin. As the carbon dioxide is expelled from the body through exhalation, the rushing bloodstream carries the oxygen to the body cells so that cellular metabolism can proceed.

Inhalation and exhalation have a profound physiological effect. Since so much of yoga is concerned with breathing, it is important for the student to understand some of the basic physiological dynamics involved. It is through employing various breathing techniques that the student will learn to manipulate these dynamics to his own advantage.

In yoga, respiration involves four stages: inhalation, retention of breath, exhalation, and retention of emptiness. Inhalation and exhalation each produces a different physiological effect which can be heightened by retention. The yoga breath begins with exhalation. In exhalation the parasympathetic nervous system is stimulated while the sympathetic nervous system relaxes, causing in turn the relaxation of internal organs, expansion of the blood vessels, and lowering of blood pressure. Peristalsis of the entire digestive tract intensifies considerably, the bladder relaxes, and secretions of the pancreas are stimulated. With inhalation the sympathetic nervous system is stimulated, resulting in an increase of blood pressure and a decrease of peristalsis. Secretions from the pancreas momentarily diminish and the bladder contracts. But the most pronounced influences of exhalation and inhalation are felt by the cardiovascular system, which, like the rest of the body, "breathes with the breather." Certain Chinese "healing breaths," which are described in chapter 5, are based on these and other physiological reactions to inhalation and exhalation.

In the process of respiration, the sound known in Indian yoga as the "mantra of health" is produced. The closest approximation of this sound is the whispered word *so* for inhalation and the whispered word *hum* for exhalation. This mantra of health is produced by partly closing the glottis at the back of the throat. Many children, youths, and healthy adults produce this mantra spontaneously while relaxing or fast asleep.

I remarked earlier that what today is considered as the "metaphysics" of breathing in Eastern thought could eventually become part of our scientific heritage and that the metaphysics of breathing, as they are understood in yoga, are based on the theory of cosmic energy, or life force, in the air. This force has not yet been detected scientifically. Perhaps the closest scientific description of this energy occurred when some Russian scientists detected minute particles of electricity called ions in the air. They also studied "rarefied air" during and after violent electrical storms. We all know how beautiful it is to breathe air that has been charged and purified in this manner. It is an experience of exhilaration, of physical and mental stimulation and accentuated well-being, as if every molecule of the body has been toned up by this ionized air. In other experiments simulated ionized air has proved helpful in treating patients suffering from maladies related to the respiratory system.

I also referred earlier to certain places on our planet where longevity is prevalent among the inhabitants. The air in these places seems to possess a particularly powerful energy charge, as if it contained far greater amounts of life force than air in other places. Science still teaches us very little about the complex effects of the air we breathe on our physical system, but the question is beginning to receive attention.

We do know that our intake of oxygen purifies our bloodstream and revitalizes every cell of the body. Our nostrils contain an intricate system of nerves that branch into the upper cortex of the brain and connect to the nervous ganglia that run along the spine. It is not difficult to accept the yoga principle of pranic energy when we consider the enormous benefits of deep breathing on the body, mind, and spirit.

The student of breath control must accept the pranic theory and train himself to believe that through various breathing exercises he can control the flow of *prana* into his system, directing it to any part of his body and thus increasing his vitality and recognizing the truth of the proverb "To control breath is to control life itself."

Experiments in America have shown that elderly people, when given increased amounts of oxygen, improve health dramatically. The basic principle of rejuvenation through improved breathing specifies the frequent use of the full abdominal yoga breath. If the student will train himself or herself to breathe a complete yoga breath while relaxing, walking, meditating, or even sleeping, the aging process can be first delayed and then, to a significant extent, reversed.

5

The Importance
of Correct Breathing

I will never forget my first breathing lesson. I was told by my teacher to go to bed early the night before and to meet him the next morning in the inner courtyard of the ashram. The ashram was located on the very top of a tiny atoll in the blue-green Chinese South Sea. The inner courtyard was surrounded by walls on three sides, while the fourth side was open, facing eastward toward a magnificent expanse of open water. In front the ground dropped hundreds of feet and, looking down, I saw the waves so far below that I couldn't hear them beating on the ancient rocks of the island.

I had been told to be ready for my lesson just before sunrise. I was also told to prepare for the lesson by carefully washing my nostrils with warm, salted water. My teacher explained to me how to do it. First, the right nostril and then the left one is held closed while the water is slowly drawn through the open nostril until it starts to flow out through the mouth. This procedure to cleanse the nasal passages was considered very important.

I was sitting quietly, looking across the water, daydreaming and wondering what I was about to experience. The teacher soon appeared. We greeted each other in the traditional manner, pressing our arms together in front of our chests and bowing from the waist while continuing to look into each other's eyes. Then we sat down side by side. He instructed me to wait until the first rays of sun reached my face and then to inhale a deep breath, retaining it for six heartbeats before exhaling. He told me that one of the ancient teachings on breathing is the marriage of two energies: The energy of the air and the energy of sunlight are "married" at the moment of sunrise. He told me with a soft smile that out of this marriage the seed of life is born and that to breathe morning air penetrated by sunlight is to breathe the very breath of life. He instructed me to breathe with my eyes closed, facing the sun until it was fully above the line of the horizon. That took about ten slow and deep breaths. He also told me to be conscious of my nostrils. There, he said, you will feel the life force.

In a short while, as if emerging from underneath the ocean, the sun started to appear. I inhaled, retained the air for six heartbeats, and then slowly exhaled. I made an inner effort to concentrate on the meaning of breathing. I felt great joy and exhilaration from this experience, and I did sense the life force in my nostrils; it was indeed in the air, distinctly separate from everything else.

That morning I was told many wonderful things about breathing. I was told that when you establish rhythmical breathing so that the length of inhalation and exhalation is equal, you are uniting yourself with the rhythm of the entire universe, which can be described as the rhythm of a pendulum. To create this rhythm I was instructed to put the middle finger of my right hand on the wrist of my left, counting six pulse beats for inhalation and six for exhalation. I breathed in this manner for quite some time and soon came to a profound inner peace and a sense of oneness with the world around me.

My next exercise was to continue rhythmical breathing while concentrating on the elusive, subtle moment at which inhalation becomes exhalation. It was this teacher who told me that inhalation represents life—the first breath of a newborn child—while exhalation signifies death—the last expiration of a dying man. The point where inhalation becomes exhalation symbolizes immortality. Concentrating on this point leads to the personal realization of the immortality of the spirit, an insight which comes to the student as direct truth.

The memory of that morning stands very clear in my mind. Then and there I realized that control of breath is not merely control of inhalation and exhalation but control of the life force. I stayed almost a year in this ashram, learning from its master many breathing techniques and gaining insights into what is perhaps the greatest secret of life.

Breath control, or *pranayama*, constitutes the fourth step of Hatha yoga. It follows the study of *asanas*, or bodily postures (these will be described as the exercises are presented). In the context of delaying aging, the study of breath control is of primary importance. The breathing exercises in this chapter will be presented on three levels: beginning, intermediate, and advanced. A beginner must first learn how to breathe with the help of the diaphragm (full abdominal breathing). He must become aware of the life force, or *prana*, in the air and acquire the personal experience of moving that energy through the body by concentrated thought. Then he can proceed to the intermediate level, which requires deeper concentration and more knowledge of the mechanics of breathing. Some of the breathing exercises are extremely complicated and should be attempted only after levels 1 and 2 are mastered.

Certain of these exercises which I cite below have, to

my best knowledge, never before been described to a Western audience. They include building of "energy fields" in the body, transmutation of various energies, and readjustment of the psyche to higher levels of consciousness. They also provide methods to activate the psychic, or nervous, centers called chakras in Indian yoga. A number of breath controls related to the "serpent energy" of Kundalini yoga will be presented, along with healing breath practices of Chinese, Indian, and Tibetan yogas.

According to tradition, a true seeker can achieve four attainments through breath control: pacification of the mind and the entire nervous system (as well as moving onto a higher plane of consciousness), building up energy, cooling the body when it is hot, warming the body when it is cold. All these breathing techniques are directly related to rejuvenation and extension of the life span, inasmuch as they purify the bloodstream and build a surplus of energy.

Preliminary Exercises

Before describing the breathing exercises, which can be done either lying prone or supine, standing, or sitting, I will indicate the variety of seated postures, or *asanas,* available to the student. There is a fascinating theory that the physical as well as the spiritual division of East and West can be traced to the different manners of sitting practiced in the two hemispheres. In the East, especially India, for thousands of years people have grown used to sitting cross-legged on the floor, a position that they believe promotes inner peace and serenity and is conducive to contemplative and meditative practices. In the cross-legged position, the entire body is physically compact and concentrated. In the West people rarely sit on the floor. We have instead a history of benches, chairs, sofas, and stools. This manner of sitting always on some type of furniture promotes unrest and stirs people to action, according to the theory I am describing. That is why the Eastern world has been called a "world of thoughts" while the Western world has been designated a "world of action." If this theory is correct, we can see what a tremendous difference these variant practices over centuries have created in the psyche as well as in the way of life. Some parts of the East are still in meditative slumber, with their way of life much as it was 2,000 years ago. In the Western world, there is a sophisticated technology that is far superior to that of the Eastern world. However, if we consider the knowledge of the inner man, the complex structure of a man on the metaphysical level, the East has progressed far ahead of the West. Only now is an exchange of values taking place between the two hemispheres. One of the most important influences of East on West may be in the manner of sitting.

Postures

There are four traditional cross-legged sitting positions in yoga which will be referred to in the exercises described hereafter. In all these poses, the back and neck should be kept in a straight line.

1. *Easy Pose (Sukhasana)*

This is a simple cross-legged position not unlike that of the European tailor. Both legs are crossed, with the ankles touching each other and the hands lightly resting on the knees. This position is usually adopted by beginners with stiff hip joints and an inability to arrange their legs in any other cross-legged position. It can be used for meditation and breathing exercises as well as for eye and neck exercises.

2. *Free Pose (Samasana)*

Another easy position for the beginner differs from the first one by the position of the ankles, which are not crossed. In the free pose, the left heel is brought close to the body at the *yoni* place (space between the anus and the sex organs) while the right foot is placed in front of it in a free attitude. This position may be slightly more difficult than the first one, but it has an advantage: Sitting in this attitude, a gentle pressure, exerted by the weight of the legs unsupported by each other, is put on the hip joints, promoting suppleness.

3. *Pose of an Adept, Pose of Attainment, Pose of Sidha (One Who Attains Inner Powers)*

This pose has a variety of names. In traditional literature it is known as *Sidha Asana.* In this pose the left heel is brought close to the *yoni* place while the right foot is placed between left calf and thigh. The pose, if properly executed, is beautifully balanced. It is used for breath control, meditation, and various practices of higher yoga.

4. *Pose of the Buddha, Pose of the Lotus (Padma Asana)*

In this pose, the left foot is placed on the right thigh with the heel touching the groin, while the right foot is placed on top of the left leg with the heel also touching the groin. Both feet are turned up. Knees are in contact with the floor. One of the beneficial aspects of this posi-

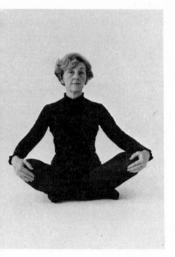

Easy Pose (*Sukhasana*)

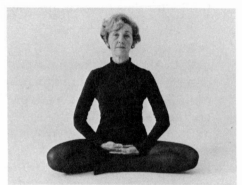

Free Pose (*Samasana*)

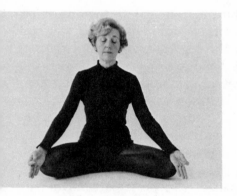

Pose of an Adept
(*Sidha Asana*)

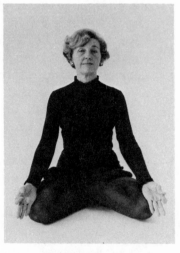

Pose of the Lotus
(*Padma Asana*)

tion, especially for contemplative and meditative practices, is that the interlocked feet slow to a certain extent the circulation of blood in the legs, releasing an extra flow of arterial blood to circulate in the upper part of the body. This pose supposedly has curative value, especially for diseases of the chest and abdomen.

With these postures in mind, we can move now to a description of full abdominal breathing and the "ha," or cleansing, breath, which are preliminary exercises to master before beginning the exercises in level 1.

Full Abdominal Breathing

The easiest way to learn the art of full abdominal breathing is to lie on the back with the fingertips lightly resting on the stomach. With eyes closed, pretend that you are sleeping. Slow down your breathing. With the fingertips, start to feel the movements of your diaphragm.[1] A useful variation is to lie with the legs drawn up and crossed and the arms above the head, wrists crossed behind the neck. This posture forces an expansion of the chest area and makes abdominal breathing even easier.

The yoga breath, or full abdominal breath, always begins with exhalation. The student is trained to use his diaphragm as well as his chest in such a way that the entire lungs are first emptied and then completely filled.

Inhalation can be visualized as a three-part movement which is actually performed in one smooth, continuous, wavelike motion. In the first stage of inhalation, the ab-

1. An effective method practiced now by a number of physiotherapists is to place a heavy book on the stomach so that the patient can watch it rise and fall while breathing. Some therapists working with asthmatic children have placed miniature ships on their stomachs to add interest to this process.

dominal muscles are slightly pushed forward, causing the diaphragm to become flattened so that the bottom part of the lungs automatically fills with air. Then the floating ribs (those at the bottom of the rib cage not connected to the breastbone) are expanded while the chest is lifted up. This movement draws air into the middle part of the lungs and then into the upper part. Expansion of the chest continues as the middle and upper lungs are filled. The abdomen now is drawn slightly in, as if to support the chest. Exhalation follows the reverse three-part movement. To insure a more complete emptying of the lungs, the diaphragm is contracted during the last stage of exhalation. Then the chest and abdomen return to their original relaxed position.

When the abdominal breath is mastered lying on the back, the student can learn how to breath correctly either sitting in a chair or in one of the traditional cross-legged positions with the palms of the hands resting on the side of the body and the fingertips meeting on the stomach. In the process of correct inhalation, the fingertips will glide apart, and during exhalation they will meet again.

Next, abdominal breath is mastered while lying on the right side in a natural, slightly curled attitude of sleep, the head resting on the right arm, the left arm lying on the hip or behind the back. The same breathing is practiced then on the other side. This simple exercise is extremely important, since we spend one-third of our lives in sleep.

Upon mastering the art of full abdominal breathing, one can practice breath controls both indoors and out-doors. With the incoming breath, *prana* is inhaled; with the outgoing breath, *prana* can be directed to any part of the body for stimulation and invigorating effects, or for healing. One exhales only carbon dioxide, or "used up" air.

"Ha," or Cleansing, Breath (Sigh of Relief)

Many cycles of breathing exercises should be terminated by a vigorous cleansing breath known as "ha" breath. Standing with feet apart, raise arms slowly as breath is inhaled (keep legs straight). Then drop the upper torso forward as you exhale vigorously, making a "ha" sound. Let arms hang loosely for a moment. Repeat three times.

Another form of cleansing breath can be done either in a standing or a seated position. After a deep inhalation the lips are pursed like the letter *o* and the breath is expelled in short blasts, driving out the stale air by rapidly contracting the floating ribs and the diaphragm. In a standing position, the cleansing breath can be accompanied by a vigorous rubbing of the lower ribs or tapping of the chest during exhalation to expedite the discharge of stale air.

The third method for the cleansing breath can also be done either in a standing or cross-legged sitting posture. It consists of expelling air in a vigorous, continuous stream.

Whatever method of cleansing breath is practiced, it is supported by the mental image of fatigue being expelled from the system. The "ha" breath is a sigh of relief. Many people do it naturally at the end of the day or week.

Level 1 (Beginning)

For the convenience of the student, the breathing techniques here are usually grouped in cycles of seven. Each cycle should be terminated by the "ha," or cleansing, breath.

Tranquilizing Breaths

In the context of delaying aging, the ability to bring about inner peace and tranquility is most important. One of the scourges of modern times is life-shortening tension, a condition that creates many mental as well as physical maladies. The ability to keep oneself in a state of balanced serenity prolongs the creative part of life. The simplest and most effective way to keep one's mind in perfect balance is through breath control. *Every time the rhythm of the breath is slowed down, breath becomes a powerful tranquilizer.*

In my casebook there is an example of a New York businessman, middle-aged and intelligent, who complained that he was suddenly beset with fits of uncontrollable rage. On the slightest provocation he would explode, abusing his secretary or even lashing out at a client, often with distressing results. After these outbursts he would fall into a state of deep remorse, unable to understand what was happening. He said he could always feel the onset of the rage, but he didn't know how to control it. Knowing how breath control has a tranquilizing and pacifying effect, I recommended that every time he felt tension he should inhale a deep breath, retain it for a few seconds, and slowly exhale. I told him that the deep breath would provide "food" for his nerves, and that with exhalation, all tension would leave his body. The next week he reported jubilantly that he had gained control over his temper. That was several years ago, and to my knowledge, he has continued to use breath control to handle this problem successfully.

Our nervous system is capable of producing a certain amount of extra energy with the purpose of activating our systems in times of emergency.We should not waste this vital energy. People spend millions of dollars on tranquilizing drugs without realizing that one of the great secrets of pacification is in breath control. Techniques of breath control can help us to keep calm in social and domestic upsets and under the stresses of work requirements and traffic snarls.

The basic principle of the tranquilizing breath controls is to slow down the rhythm of the breath. Normally, we breathe from fifteen to twenty times a minute, but through the pacifying breaths this rhythm is lowered to four or five breaths per minute. Certain exercises slow the rhythm of the breath to as few as two breaths per minute. All these exercises pacify the nervous system.

EXERCISE 1: The Pendulum Breath
     Position: Cross-legged, back and neck in a straight line, hands resting on knees.
     Breath: Slow breath to 6 heartbeats per inhalation and 6 per exhalation (this will slow the rhythm of the breath to only 5 breaths per minute), creating the rhythm of a pendulum.
     Duration: Five to ten minutes of this breathing will produce a pacifying effect on the mind and the entire nervous system.

EXERCISE 2: Variation of Pendulum Breath
     Same as above, but with mind concentrated on the image of peaceful and beautiful scenery.

EXERCISE 3: *Om* Breath
     Same as above, but the slow rhythm of this breath is broken by retention of the inhalation sufficiently long to pronounce silently the mantra *om*.

EXERCISE 4: Gentle Breathing
     Position: Cross-legged, back and neck in a straight line, hands resting on knees.

Breath: Slow down the rhythm of the breath as much as possible and, at the same time, observe perfect quietness of inhalation and exhalation.

Remarks: Gentle breathing stands out as one of the most powerful pacifiers of the mind. Very often it is used in meditation because of its power to bring about inner peace and tranquility. Often in the Eastern ashrams, to test the ability of the student to breathe the gentle breath correctly, a lighted candle is brought close to the face of the student, who is instructed to perform the complete inhalation and exhalation so gently that the flame of the candle is not moved.

EXERCISE 5: Center of Peace
    Position: Cross-legged.
    Breath: Slow rhythm.
    Meditation: The student forms a mental image of the life force directed to the back of the head in the area of the medulla oblongata.
    Remarks: It has long been noted that concentration on certain centers of the body can produce a pacifying and tranquilizing effect. A pacifying effect can be achieved in a remarkably short time with this breath.

EXERCISE 6: Purifier of the Mind
    Position: Cross-legged.
    Breath: Slow rhythm.
    Meditation: A mental image is formed in which *prana* is directed to the head, gradually banishing all thoughts, bringing about stillness of the mind.
    Remarks: Research on the human mind today suggests that about 100 thoughts, many of them negative in essence, pass through the human mind every minute. This continuous mental chattering is one of the main causes of our mental unrest. This exercise can help to turn *dis*-ease into ease (or health).

EXERCISE 7: Breath of Unification

Position: This exercise can be practiced either in a sitting or a supine position and usually is done outdoors if weather permits.

Breath: Slow rhythm.

Meditation: The student forms a mental image that his entire body is taking part in the breathing. He is slowly merging with his breath.

Energizing Breaths

Chronic fatigue is one of the phenomena of modern times. It seems to me that fatigue is not determined by age—everyone is tired. I am certain that a major cause of fatigue is faulty breathing. Fatigue is sometimes explained as the result of the accumulation of lactic acid in the bloodstream. Normally, this acid is discharged through a night of good sleep. Often, however, in cases of poor breathing, a residue of tiredness is carried into the next day and the next. This cumulative effect of fatigue can be corrected by regular breathing exercises designed to build energy.

The uniting principle of all these energizing breaths is the belief that we can separate pranic force from the air and direct it to any part of the body by an effort of the will and by concentration. A thought is actually a directing power, and in most cases, the ultimate success of the student is proportional to the quality of concentration. If the right concentration is maintained throughout practice, success is always achieved, but if the mind wanders, the entire "magic" of the practice is broken (in the Tibetan tradition, human concentration is considered to be magic).

Indian yogis accept the solar plexus *(Manipura* chakra) as the focus for pranic energy; a great number of breathing exercises have that part of the body as the point of concentration. A student is taught to imagine that with the incoming breath, he is drawing *prana* into his system and directing it to the solar plexus, whereas with the outgoing breath, he exhales only the used air. The breathing exercises related to the solar plexus can be done in sitting positions or on one's back, as well as while walking. Below is a set of energy-charging exercises suitable for the beginner. *In each of these, the student forms a mental image of directing* prana *to the solar plexus.*

Standing Position: Quiet Cycle

EXERCISE 1
     Breath: A complete breath is inhaled and retained as long as comfortable. The image is formed during the slow exhalation.

EXERCISE 2
     Breath and Movement: After deep inhalation, both arms are raised above the head, palms together. Breath is again retained and slowly exhaled.

EXERCISE 3
     Breath and Movement: After full breath is inhaled, palms are pressed in front of the chest in the attitude of prayer. Retention and exhalation as above.

EXERCISE 4
     Breath and Movement: The two previous movements are combined while full breath is inhaled. Arms are raised, palms brought together, then slowly lowered to position in front of the chest. Then breath is exhaled.

EXERCISE 5

Breath and Movement: Breath is inhaled, then arms are raised. While breath is retained, the trunk is slowly bent to the right and then to the left. Then breath is exhaled.

EXERCISE 6

Breath and Movement: Inhale, rise onto the tip of your toes, retain breath in this attitude, then bring heels down while you exhale.

EXERCISE 7

Breath and Movement: Inhale, retain breath while tensing every muscle of the body. Relax, exhale, and direct *prana* to the solar plexus.

Standing Position: Vigorous Cycle (Mouth Breathing)

EXERCISE 1

Breath and Movement: Inhale a full breath while stretching arms forward (parallel) to shoulder level. While retaining breath, vigorously swing arms apart to the sides, then together in front, then apart to sides, together, apart, together. Exhale and drop arms by sides. (Remember in all these exercises to direct *prana* to the solar plexus.)

EXERCISE 2

Breath and Movement: Inhale. Retain breath and vigorously swing the arms forward and up over the head, down, up, down, up, down. Exhale and relax.

EXERCISE 3

Breath and Movement: Inhale. Lock the breath by closing the glottis and swing arms like windmills, twice forward and upward, crossing in front of the chest. Then reverse the movement, bringing arms down, crossing in front of the chest. Exhale and relax.

EXERCISE 4

Breath and Movement: Inhale. Stretch arms forward, retain breath, then pull arms back against shoulders with a vigorous movement that shakes the whole body. Stretch forward, pull back, forward, back. Exhale.

EXERCISE 5

Breath and Movement: Inhale. Bend upper body to left, vigorously swinging arms up from sides to cross over the head, then down; then perform the same movement to the right. Exhale.

EXERCISE 6

Breath and Movement: Inhale. Retain breath. Vigorously massage and slightly squeeze the floating ribs with the palms. Exhale.

EXERCISE 7

Breath and Movement: Inhale and retain breath. Gently tap the chest with the fingers. Exhale in powerful short gusts, pursing the lips like the letter *o.*

Sitting Position

Any of the traditional cross-legged positions described previously are suitable for these exercises. The neck and back should be kept in a straight line, with hands resting on the knees. During retention of breath, form the mental image of *prana* being separated from the air and directed to the solar plexus to be stored there. Keep this image during exhalation.

EXERCISE 1

Breath: Deep and rhythmical. After a few minutes, break the rhythm by retaining the full breath for 3 heart-beats.

Repetitions: Twelve slow, deep, rhythmical breaths are sufficient to feel the sensation of increased vitality, if the concentration is not disturbed throughout the practice.

EXERCISE 2

As above, but with arms relaxed and fingers inter-laced in front of the body.

EXERCISE 3

As above, but with hands pressed in front of the chest in the attitude of prayer. After deep inhalation, palms are pressed against each other with considerable force for the duration of 1 heartbeat.

EXERCISE 4

As above, but with hands (interlaced fingers) resting on top of the head. Inhale, raising the arms up with the palms away from the body. Breath is retained for 3 heart-beats. With exhalation, palms return to original position.

Supine Position

EXERCISE 1

Breath and Movement: Hands under neck, head and shoulders are raised off the floor while full breath is in-haled. Return to original position, exhale. During exhala-tion, one creates the image of *prana* being directed to and retained in the solar plexus.

EXERCISE 2

As above, but lift up both legs in the process of inhalation. Retain for a moment, lower legs, exhale.

EXERCISE 3

Breath and Movement: Hands under neck, feet flat on floor, breath is inhaled while hips are raised until muscles of buttocks become tensed. After brief retention, the body is lowered to the original position, breath exhaled.

EXERCISE 4

Breath and Movement: Hands alongside body, chest is raised up so that shoulder blades are clear of floor. After retaining breath for a few seconds, return to original position and exhale.

Benefit: This exercise is exceptionally beneficial for people with bad posture or round shoulders. It also increases the capacity of the chest. Very often it is given by physiotherapists to people with breathing problems.

EXERCISE 5

Breath and Movement: With inhalation, breath retained, move legs in scissors movement as many times as comfortable. Exhale. Lower legs.

EXERCISE 6

As above, but instead of scissors, describe a few circles with legs.

EXERCISE 7

Breath and Movement: Lying flat on back, knees brought close to stomach, deeply inhale, stretch legs up at right angle to body; then allow legs to relax completely and drop to original position. Exhale.

Repetitions: Each of these exercises can be done as many times as one feels comfortable with full concentration and correct breathing.

Level 2 (Intermediate)

When the experience of controlling *prana* has been acquired, concentration improved, and power of imagination developed, breathing exercises on the intermediate level can be started.

Pacifying Breaths

Standing Position

EXERCISE 1: Nine Tranquilizing Breaths
     A. Breath and Movement: A very slow breath is inhaled while both arms are brought forward and raised parallel above the head. Exhale while causing the arms to describe a circle, palms toward floor, until arms again are alongside the body.
     Meditation: The mind is concentrated on the sound of *om* and the sign of the circle.
     Repetitions: 4.
     B. Breath and Movement: Inhalation is combined with raising arms above head sideways, fingertips touching for a moment. Reverse movement as you exhale. Arms are brought down, palms toward floor.
     Meditation: Mind is concentrated on the sound *ma* and the sign of the triangle.
     Repetitions: 3.
     C. Breath and Movement: Arms are raised forward and parallel during inhalation until arms are above head. They are brought down in the same manner during exhalation.

Meditation: Mind is concentrated on the sound *pa* and the sign of parallel lines.

Repetitions: 2.

Remarks: These nine deliberate, slow breaths result in pacification of the entire nervous system and mind. During practice the mind is held between *mantra* and *yantra* (sound and sign) and remains calm. The exercise requires a well-developed power of concentration and imagination.

Seated Position

EXERCISE 2: *Anahata* Breath

Position: Any of the traditional cross-legged positions described above are suitable. Back and neck in a straight line. Mouth relaxed (be sure teeth are not clenched).

Breath: Deep and rhythmical.

Meditation: Concentration is on the point in the middle of the chest known as the cardiac plexus, or *Anahata* chakra. Direct the stream of life force to this chakra.

Benefit: This breathing brings peace and tranquility to the mind through slowing down the personal time clock, or the rhythm of the heart, and lowering the blood pressure.

EXERCISE 3: *Ajna* Chakra

As above, but with eyes closed and rolled upward. *Prana* is directed between the eyebrows to the *Ajna* chakra. The benefit is a sensation of mental peace and enlightenment.

EXERCISE 4: *Rechaka* Breath

As above, but emphasis is placed on exhalation *(rechaka),* eventually prolonging exhalation into emptiness. The duration is 5 minutes, and the benefit is pacification of the nervous system and lowering of the blood pressure.

EXERCISE 5: Stillness of the Mind

As above, but during the meditation all thoughts should be eliminated gradually, aiming at stillness of the mind. Even 60 seconds of complete stillness is a wonderful pacifier of the mind and nervous system.

EXERCISE 6: Breathing with the Bones of the Body

Form an image that you are inhaling and exhaling through the bones first of the legs, then of the arms, chest, and eventually of the skull. If done with concentration, this exercise has the remarkable power of producing a sensation of physical well-being and energy. It requires a real feeling of cosmic energy and a well-developed power of imagination.

EXERCISE 7: Yoga *Nidra* (to be practiced while on one's back)

Form an image that you are merging your body with the air in this order: the right leg, left arm, left leg, right arm, and then the rest of the body. Imagine that you have become invisible, at one with the air. The sensation of lightness and bodilessness leads to profound relaxation and complete recharging of the entire system in a short time. Among *nidras,* which are techniques for relaxing and energizing the body, the *nidra* of mergence is one of the easiest and most popular in yoga. Its effect is based on the power of imagination.

Energy-Charging Exercises

Seated Position

EXERCISE 1

Position: Any traditional cross-legged position.
Breath: Inhale deeply, tense muscles of the body,

retain breath for a few seconds. Exhale.

Meditation: Form mental image of the life force directed to every cell of the body.

Repetitions: 12 slow breaths.

EXERCISE 2

Position: Traditionally, this exercise is performed in the lotus position.

Breath and Movement: After deep inhalation, palms are placed on the floor at the sides. While breath is retained, the whole body is lifted up. The body is slowly lowered as breath is exhaled.

Meditation: Consciousness is directed to accumulating *prana* in the solar plexus.

Repetitions: 6 breaths.

EXERCISE 3

Position: Lotus.

Breath and Movement: Inhale, raise body. This time, instead of holding this position, drop to the floor so that the body shakes gently. Repeat 2 or 3 times before exhaling.

Meditation: Concentrate on the thought that each body cell is being recharged and purified with *prana*.[2]

Repetitions: 4.

EXERCISE 4

Position: Any traditional cross-legged posture. The easy cross-legged pose could be substituted for the pose of the lotus.

Breath and Movement: Place hands behind the neck, fingers interlaced, while thumbs are placed behind the ears at the sides of the neck. With each inhalation, breath

2. With added *bandhas* this exercise will be a *mudra* of perforation (pp. 83–84).

is retained for a few seconds. A gentle but firm pressure is created by the thumbs in the region of the jugular vein, resulting in an increase of the blood pressure.

Meditation: Concentrate on the thought that the bloodstream is becoming charged with *prana*.

Repetitions: 4.

EXERCISE 5

Position: Lotus, if possible.

Breath and Movement: Inhale full breath and, while breath is retained, lower body backward in supine position. After retaining breath for 4–6 heartbeats, raise upper body and exhale.

Meditation: While breath is retained, mind is concentrated on the thought of building up energy in the solar plexus.

Repetitions: 4–6.

EXERCISE 6

Position: Lotus, if possible.

Breath and Movement: Inhale and lean backward, resting on forearms and elbows while locked legs are raised at the same angle as the body. Breath is retained as long as comfortable and then one resumes original position. Exhale.

Meditation: Same as above.

Repetitions: 3.

Remarks: This pose is known as the "scale" pose *(tulungasana)* and is a powerful method for building a surplus of *prana* in the solar plexus.

EXERCISE 7

Same as above, but forming the mental image that with incoming breath *prana* is inhaled and with outgoing breath it is directed to every cell of the body.

Duration: 5 minutes.

Supine Position

EXERCISE 1: Breathing Away Fatigue

Breath and Meditation: In a completely relaxed attitude, deep and rhythmical breath established, the student concentrates on the thought that with each exhaled breath he is directing *prana* through millions of pores of the skin, thus breathing away tiredness.

Duration: Five minutes of this exercise is usually sufficient to experience the sensation of being refreshed.

EXERCISE 2

Same as above, but with fingertips placed on the solar plexus. An image is formed that the life force flows through the fingertips and is redirected to its customary seat in the body.[3]

Duration: 5–10 minutes.

EXERCISE 3

Breath and Movement: Lying in a relaxed position, a deep breath is inhaled and the body is stretched while breath is retained. Relax with exhalation.

Repetitions: 6.

EXERCISE 4

Breath and Movement: Inhale a deep breath and raise the knees until they are pressed against the abdomen. The hands are clasped around the knees. Exhale, release the hands, and lower the legs.

Repetitions: 4.

Remarks: This form of breath control is not advisable

---

3. Kirlian photography has established the existence of fields of energy around our fingertips. This is another example of science verifying ancient ideas. Often, pictures of yogis in old texts have shown them painted with rays of light emanating from their fingertips.

in cases of high blood pressure since it builds up pressure in the head, flushing the face and head with a supply of richly oxygenated arterial blood. For this reason, it is used as a rejuvenating and beautifying exercise as well as an energy-charging one.[4]

EXERCISE 5

Breath and Meditation: Lying completely relaxed, deep rhythmical breath established, *prana* is directed to the roots of spinal nerves with each exhalation. Full concentration brings the sensation of warmth and refreshment.

Duration: 5 minutes.

EXERCISE 6

Breath and Movement: This exercise is based on alternately tensing and relaxing the entire body. Lying on one's back, with feet and arms apart, one achieves complete relaxation by an effort of will. With a deep inhalation, the legs and arms as well as head and trunk are raised, leaving only the buttocks in contact with the floor. Every muscle of the body is deliberately tensed. The pose is retained for a few seconds, and then the original relaxed attitude is regained.

Remarks: This exercise causes the "ebb and tide" of the rich arterial blood to every muscle group in the body, nourishing, toning up, and revitalizing the entire system.

EXERCISE 7

Closely related to the above exercise is the balancing–energizing pose.

---

4. In variation of this exercise, knees are pressed to the stomach and position retained while breathing normally for one or two minutes. This technique is known as "gas squeezer."

Breath and Movement: In the supine position, knees drawn up to the stomach while fingertips of both hands are touching at the middle of the chest *(Anahata* chakra), one inhales a deep breath. The legs are stretched at a 45-degree angle and the body is raised up in a **V** pose with the arms spread apart. Breath and balance are retained for 3 heartbeats, then the original relaxed position is resumed. The life force is directed to the solar plexus during exhalation.

Repetitions: 4–6.

Each of the above exercises can be practiced as many times as is comfortable, avoiding fatigue at all costs. If done in the manner prescribed they will recharge the body with energy, creating a sensation of physical and mental well-being.

Level 3 (Advanced)

Introduction

The higher aspects of breath control at times are profoundly involved and complicated, and the claims associated with them are fascinating. According to tradition, these breath controls can extend the life span to 150 years, and they can help one to grow a new skin on the face and body. As we have seen, these claims are not so preposterous as they may sound. We can find in breath control the greatest source of life, health, vitality, and rejuvenation. Before beginning these exercises, the ideas behind breath control presented earlier should be understood as much as possible so that in breathing practices the mind's power can support the physical effort.

Behind these exercises is an attempt to harness cosmic energy. When breath control has been mastered, cosmic energy is mastered, too, so that the macrocosm of the universe is united with the microcosm of the body. The profound metaphysical formula "as above, so below" is at the center of these teachings. Breath control leads to control of consciousness. No longer bound by the limitations of the physical body, a person can perceive all things in their fullness, although, through the intermediary of the senses, he can know only limited fragments. Breath control is intimately related to meditative and contemplative practices. On many occasions, breath is the very object of meditation.

According to *Shivasamhita,* an ancient scripture on yoga, through breath control a student could gain supernatural powers, "cross beyond the ocean of sin and virtue, and freely wander in three worlds." Not only the present and the past but the future become a part of the person's awareness. There is also the warning, however, that acquired superhuman powers, if used for personal gain, will destroy the practitioner.

Many higher-level breath control practices have been clothed in secret to make them unavailable for unprepared persons. With the help of yoga scholars I have managed to decode most of the *pranayamas* that are well known among yoga adepts. Alongside the traditional *pranayamas* of Indian yoga exist many techniques of breathing from Chinese and Tibetan schools. In the past many remote ashrams, retreats, and monasteries of these countries were famous for their breath controls. The techniques were closely guarded and disclosed only to trusted seekers. I have been privileged to learn some of these unusual breath controls which, to the best of my knowledge, have never been revealed to the Western world. Even in the Eastern world, they are known to a very limited number of people. Of the ones presented below, I have checked my findings with the masters of three yogas. Satisfied with the results, I present them in a form that I consider suitable for the Western student.

Preliminary Exercises: Alternating Nostrils, *Mudras, Bandhas*

Alternating Nostrils

One of the generally unknown phenomena of breathing is that everyone tends to favor one nostril or the other; indeed, these long, winding nasal passages can't be exactly the same. A simple test can establish in a few minutes which is the dominant nostril, or the nostril through which it is "easier" for one to breathe: Seated in any of the traditional cross-legged positions, the left nostril is closed first. One breathes quickly in and out through the right nostril with an inward "rubbing" motion of the breath. After half a dozen in and out breaths, change nostrils. Repeat the exercise 6 times. In most cases you will be able to distinguish which nostril feels more open for the breath.[5]

Nature has its mysterious law of alternating breath many times during a twenty-four-hour period. Schools of yoga are divided in stipulating how many times, but they agree that the breath flows equally through both nostrils only for a short period twice a day, at midday and at midnight. These are both considered dangerous periods. In this context, the traditional belief to a certain extent corresponds to the Chinese Confucian text, the *I Ching,* wherein one is taught that balance is always followed by imbalance. One of the metaphysical explanations of this phenomenon is that at the primitive stage of man's development, nature forbids him to control the flow of cosmic energy into his system. Only those who

5. According to the Tantric tradition, women with a dominant right nostril in most cases produce male offspring as a first child, whereas women with a dominant left nostril give birth first to girls. Many practicers of Tantra yoga suggest blocking the unfavored nostril during copulation to influence the sex of the child.

make themselves ready by spiritual attainment are able to achieve this control.

It is also taught that during sleep, if we are resting on the right side, breath flows easily through the left nostril (cooling nostril); sleeping on the left side causes breath to flow easily through the right nostril (warming nostril). Often, the sensing of heat or chill in the body could be accounted for by this theory. Sleeping too long on the right side, for instance, brings chill. Over a period of years I have conducted my own survey of this theory, asking my students to note on what side they were lying when they awoke feeling cold or hot. The testimonies tended to verify the theory.

It is believed in yoga that the nervous centers in the brain are stimulated only by breathing through the nostrils (not the mouth). If this theory is correct, many cases of child idiocy or mental retardation could be traced to blockage in nostrils and consequent breathing through the mouth. The typical image of the village idiot always shows a profusely salivating, half-open mouth. At the opposite end of the spectrum, certain breathing exercises of Raja yoga are practiced in order to achieve a stimulating effect on the brain, bringing about the development of one's latent mental powers.

According to yoga theory, *ida* and *pingala*,[6] after they ascend to the *Brahma* chakra, or top of the head, descend to the medulla oblongata, then down the spinal column, forming the main ganglia of the sympathetic nervous system. Thus, not only the brain but the entire sympathetic nervous system is stimulated in the act of nostril breathing. Many breathing exercises that involve breath through alternate nostrils are based on this theory.

A student of higher breath controls could learn in a

6. Mentioned during discussion of the metaphysics of breath (chap. 4).

fairly short space of time the art of alternating the flow of breath through the right and left nostrils. By an effort of will one can learn how to make breath flow readily through the right or left nostril, according to one's concentration.

Mudras

Many Indian *pranayamas* are practiced in conjunction with *mudras,*[7] or locks. Frequently, the advanced breathing techniques require a *hand mudra,* which is a special position of the fingers of the right hand. In the Indian tradition, the hand is opened, then the index finger and middle finger are brought down to the palm. The hand is brought to the nose. Closing and opening the right and left nostrils is done with the thumb for the right nostril and the ring finger for the left nostril. In the Chinese tradition, only the index finger is brought down to the palm, and the thumb and middle finger are used. Some Western people have difficulty arranging fingers in the prescribed manner. A number of *pranayamas* in China and Tibet use only the index finger and thumb. One can choose from these positions. These *hand mudras* are also referred to as *mudras of breath control.*

Another *hand mudra* often used in yoga exercises is called the *mudra of knowledge.* Here, one bends the index finger down to touch the thumb while holding the other fingers straight. The hands are then rested on the knees while one is seated cross-legged. This *mudra* serves as a reminder to the practitioner that he is conscious of what he is doing.

The *Maha mudra,* also known as the "great *mudra*"

7. The word *mudra* means "to lock" or "to seal." Traditional texts mention twenty-five mudras. The most important and suitable for Western students are described in this chapter.

or "arch gesture," is a powerful body technique that is specifically beneficial for the brain because of its "flushing" effect. *People with high blood pressure should never attempt to do it.* Sitting on a mat, the right leg is stretched forward, while the heel of the left foot is pressed to the *yoni* place. After leaning forward, put the forehead to the knee and grasp the sole of the right foot with both hands. Inhale a full breath and press the chin to the chest. At the same time, tense the rectum, drawing it upward. The position is retained for 6 heartbeats, or as long as comfortable. Then breath is exhaled and the body is returned to the original position. Reverse the position of the legs and repeat. The *Maha mudra* creates a powerful inrush of arterial blood to the brain and vital glands in the upper part of the body. This *mudra* is so potent that no more than 6 repetitions is suggested at one sitting.

Shivasamhita speaks very highly of this practice and lists these benefits: "The fire of digestion will flare up and all diseases will be destroyed. The body will have a marvellous brilliance. Together with old age, death will be defeated and desired results easily gained. The senses will be controlled." The manner of prescribed breathing varies among schools of yoga, but the technique described above is frequently used.

The *Shanmukhi mudra,* sometimes known as the "ten-fingered gesture," is practiced as a means of stilling the mind and revitalizing the five senses. It is an attempt to switch off the mind from the influence of the senses in order to attain a state of pure consciousness. It is believed that during retention of the breath, the senses are revitalized by cosmic energy, while during exhalation, they are completely rested, resulting in profound mental relaxation as well.

Seated cross-legged, inhale through both nostrils and bring the chin to the chest and lock it there. Ears are closed with the thumbs, eyes with the tips of the index fingers, nostrils with the middle fingers, while the mouth is touched by the fourth finger of each hand. The little fingers are in the air, symbolizing relaxation of the sense of touch. In that manner, breath is retained for 6–12 heartbeats and then slowly exhaled through both nostrils, while the chin is raised. The chin is again locked at the end of exhalation, with the emptiness of the lungs retained as long as comfortable. It is believed that after regular practice of this *mudra,* one can see better, smell better, hear better, taste better, and can develop a more delicate sense of touch.

The *Yoga mudra* is sometimes known as the symbol of yoga. It is another powerful technique designed to stimulate the brain and awaken latent forces in the *ajna* chakra. Traditionally, it is performed on a comfortable mat in the lotus position. With hands clasped behind the back (one hand holding the other wrist), inhale, bend forward until the head touches the floor. Retain the breath as long as comfortable, then exhale as you come up. *People with high blood pressure should not attempt this exercise or the next one.*

Pavanamukasana mudra flushes the head with blood. To perform it, lie on the back with arms by the sides. Inhale, drawing up the legs, and press the knees against the stomach with the hands while breath is retained. Release breath and lower legs.

Mahavedha mudra (the great perforation). Sit in the lotus position, inhale full breath, place both arms on the floor, and raise the body while breath is retained. Drop the body gently to the floor. Repeat 2 or 3 times and exhale. During the movement, chin is locked to the chest, and rectum contracted. This is a very important *mudra,* which, according to *Shivasamhita,* cures diseases and stops aging if practiced once every 3 hours each day.

As this is very difficult to achieve in our urban society, I recommend practice of this *mudra* 3 or 4 times along with other practices.

Prana-apana mudra is one of the most important *mudras* in the context of delaying aging and improving general health. Traditionally it is done in *sidha-asana* pose, where the left heel is brought close to the *yoni* place (space between anus and genitals) and the right foot is carefully placed between left calf and thigh, both knees as close to the floor as possible. With hands resting on the knees, deep breath is inhaled and chin locked to the chest. At the same time the anus is forcibly drawn up while navel is drawn in, as if these two parts are going to meet each other. After breath is retained for 3 heart-beats, body is relaxed, chin raised up, and breath exhaled.

Concentration in this *mudra* is on the accumulation of *prana* in the *Manipura* chakra during inhalation, while during retention of breath and 3 powerful locks (chin, anus, and navel), concentration is on transforming *prana* into *apana*[8] (cosmic energy into excretory power).

Bandhas[9]

In addition to the *mudras,* a number of muscular contractions known as *bandhas* are practiced in conjunction with breath controls. There are three main *bandhas* which must be learned thoroughly before practicing higher breath controls.

First: Mula Bandha, or Root Contraction

8. According to ancient treatises, there are ten vital energies in the physical-subtle body. Each one is associated with a physical function but is also a subtle energy. They are listed as *prana*—breathing, *apana*—excreting, *vyana*—circulation, *udana*—coughing, *samana*—digesting, *naga*—eructation, *kurma*—blinking, *krikara*—sneezing, *deva-datta*—yawning, and *dhanam-jaya*—assimilation.

9. For all practical purposes and to avoid confusion, *bandhas* and *mudras* are all the same. Often, in the traditional text, *bandhas* are described as *mudras.*

This *bandha* involves an ability to contract the muscles of the anus by drawing it inward and releasing it at will. It is not a difficult practice and can be learned by anyone in a fairly short time. It is done in the cross-legged position used during certain breathing practices. According to the teachings, it prevents vital energy from escaping the body. As the anus is the terminal point of the roots of the spinal nerves, contraction and relaxation of this part of the body bring a stimulating effect to the entire nervous system. It is one of the most important practices for prolonging the life span and youthfulness of the body. *Shivasamhita* describes this *bandha* as one which conquers old age and death.

Second: Jalandhara Bandha, or Net-holding Contraction

This *bandha* consists of pressing the chin tightly to the chest, closing the net of arteries at the neck. *Shivasamhita* speaks about this practice in allegorical language: "This *bandha* prevents the ambrosia of the thousand-petalled lotus from being devoured by digestive fire. The wise yogi comes to drink himself, gain immortality, and wander with delight through the three worlds." My interpretation is that the system of glands in the brain is powerfully stimulated in this *bandha.* An extra secretion of hormones from glands in the brain is mixed with the increased secretion of thyroid, parathyroid, saliva, and adenoid glands located in the neck. Because of chin pressure, these secretions are united in the throat rather than going straight to the stomach. Thus, by practicing this *bandha,* we are manufacturing our own "elixir of life," altering to a certain extent the chemistry of our bodies.

Third: Uddiyan Bandha, or Flying Contraction

This *bandha* could be practiced in a sitting or a standing position. It consists of drawing abdominal muscles back to the spine and up while breath is completely exhaled. It is a powerful stimulation for digestion and elimination.

In the standing position, one places one's feet about a foot and a half apart, hands on thighs, knees slightly bent. After complete exhalation, abdominal muscles are contracted, retained in that position for a few seconds, and then relaxed. Contraction is done again and again until one feels satisfied. In any of the traditional sitting positions the method is the same, with fingers pointed inward as hands rest on knees. *This* bandha *should be practiced on an empty stomach.*

When you have mastered this part, try to learn to contract and relax quickly, making a flapping movement in and out several times before relaxing and inhaling again.

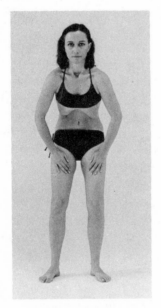

Stomach contraction
(*Uddiyan*)

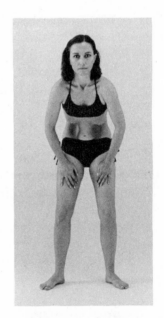

Stomach contraction
(*Nauli*)

Fourth: Nauli

This exercise involves a more elaborate control of the abdominal muscles. Inhale, exhale, and draw back the stomach as described in *uddiyan,* above. Then make a downward thrusting contraction at the pit of the stomach, the base of the abdominal recti muscles. The muscles will respond by firming into a hard column up the center of the abdomen (see illustration). This contraction should be practiced until you can see the column. Then try the same procedure on the right side and the left of the abdomen, in each case forming a hard ridge with the rest of the abdomen hollow. After you have learned to make these separations, practice contracting them one after the other, quickly, in a rotating, wavelike motion across the stomach: center to right, center to left, and so on, in a continuous movement. This movement produces a deep and powerful massage of every vital organ in the abdomen; it helps to correct disorders related to constipation, indigestion, and menstruation.

Regular Pranayamas[10]

Note: Most *pranayamas* are practiced with the eyes closed for better concentration.

EXERCISE 1: Regular *Pranayama*

Seated cross-legged, back and neck in a straight line, hands in *mudra of knowledge,* and mind pacified by rhythmical breathing, with index finger pressed to palm, raise the right hand to the nose. Pressing the right nostril with the thumb, inhale through the left nostril, counting 6 heartbeats. Exhale through the right nostril for the same time. Immediately afterward, breath is inhaled through

---

10. Any conscious interruption of normal breathing is *pranayama.*

the right nostril and exhaled through the left nostril. In *regular pranayama,* the breath flows in a perfectly regimented manner through the right and left nostrils. The student is conscious that both *nadis* (*ida* and *pingala*) are equally stimulated. This *pranayama* is practiced only for a short period of time. It is considered a preliminary exercise to more complicated breath controls.

EXERCISE 2: *Pranayama* of Energy
    Positioned as above, inhale through the right nostril, counting 6 heartbeats. Both nostrils are closed, using the ring finger and thumb, chin locked. Breath is retained for the duration of 6 heartbeats. Exhale through left nostril to the ratio of 12 heartbeats. Repeat procedure in reverse. During retention of breath, concentrate on the *Manipura* chakra, the seat of energy in the body.

EXERCISE 3: Classical *Pranayama*
    This *pranayama* has a particular rhythm of inhalation, retention, exhalation. Seated in a cross-legged position, draw breath in through left nostril to the count of 4. Press chin to chest, forming the net-holding contraction. Retain breath for 16 counts. During retention, closing of anus, or *mula bandha,* is observed. Exhale through right nostril to 8 counts. After complete exhalation, stomach is drawn up in *uddiyan bandha,* or flying contraction, which is retained as long as is comfortable. In the rhythm of this *pranayama* the counts 4, 16, 8 can be increased with practice. In advanced states, inhale to 16, retain for 64, exhale to 32. Only 12 of these *pranayamas* are suggested at the beginning, but eventually 36 can be completed at every sitting.

EXERCISE 4: *Surya Bhedana,* or Piercing of the Sun
    Any cross-legged posture is suggested for this simple but powerful technique. Inhale through the right nostril

and retain as long as is comfortable, then exhale through the same nostril. Up to 20 *pranayamas* are suggested in the beginning, with the number gradually increasing.

All textbooks suggest that this *pranayama* develops bodily heat and should be practiced during winter or in a cold climate. Tradition says that this method increases the production of bile and can cure headaches. It is also one of the techniques of the Tibetan art of *dumo,* or psychic heat.

EXERCISE 5: Awakening *Pranayama*

Seated in a cross-legged pose, right hand arranged in the *hand mudra* of breath control, the breath is quickly inhaled through the right nostril and exhaled through the left. Breathe 10 shallow, vigorous breaths, right in and left out; change to breathe in through the left and out through the right. Since it is done in a vigorous and quick manner, it should not be done longer than 3 minutes. Stimulation of *ida* and *pingala* in the left and right nostrils leads to stimulation of the entire nervous system as well as the mind.

EXERCISE 6: *Bhastrika,* or Blacksmith Bellows

This is closely related to the previous *pranayama.* Quick and vigorous inhalations and exhalations are done through both nostrils. A cycle of 6 "rubbings" terminates in deep and complete inhalation, after which lips are pursed like the letter *o* and breath is expelled in vigorous, cleansing bursts. Emphasis is on exhalation.

There is a more complicated method in Indian tradition. Seated in the lotus position (considered the best for it), breathe 10 vigorous and rapid breaths through the left nostril, followed by the eleventh deep breath through the same nostril. Retain as long as comfortable with the help of the chin lock. Exhale through the right nostril. Upon complete exhalation, the *uddiyan bandha,* or flying contraction, is executed for 4 heartbeats. The same procedure is repeated through the right nostril.

This *pranayama* is known as a blood purifier and energy instigator. It is used in cases of many diseases related to the bloodstream. Like most *pranayamas,* this one prolongs age and cures many diseases. Being a very powerful one, only 10 rounds are recommended 2 times a day, morning and evening.

EXERCISE 7: *Bhramari,* or the Bee

This exercise is known as "the bee" because it produces a gentle humming sound. It has several variations, but the most usual is done in the pose of the adept (see cross-legged positions, p. 56), with the chin locked throughout the practice. While closed eyes are focused on the point between the eyebrows, the student concentrates on the humming sound produced by the partly closed glottis while breathing deeply and rhythmically. This bee sound is another mantra of health.

EXERCISE 8: *Plavini,* or the Floating Breath Control

In the lotus position, both arms are raised straight up. Inhale through both nostrils. Then lie back (legs remain crossed) with arms clasped under the head like a pillow (left palm under right shoulder, right palm under left shoulder). Hold position as long as is comfortable (duration increasing with practice). Mind should be concentrated on the thought of lightness. Reassuming the seated position, breath is exhaled through both nostrils.

Together with the gentle breath described previously in exercises for the beginning level (p. 62), this breath control conveys the sensation of extreme lightness. An ancient treatise speaks of three attainments related to lightness that can be achieved by the serious seeker: the ability to balance on one's big toes, the ability to suspend one's bodily weight on one's fingertips, and even walking on water!

The Art of *Dumo,* or Psychic Heat

On a little plateau high up in the Himalayas, I saw five lamas engaged in a strange practice. During the beautiful and sunny days of the short Himalayan summer, they were rhythmically raising their heads to the sun, inhaling deep breaths through the right nostril, keeping the left closed with the forefinger. After the complete inhalation, both nostrils were closed and the chin locked to the chest. For a few moments, they were engaged in deep contemplation in this attitude. Their heads were then raised again to face the sun. Breath was inhaled through the right nostril, and the whole procedure was repeated again and again for at least half an hour. When they finished, with traditional humbleness I inquired what they had been doing and received a rather astonishing answer: "We have been accumulating the warmth of the sunlight in the *Manipura* chakra. It will help us to survive a long and cold winter."

This experience convinced me of the remarkable power of mind these people possessed. The image of the golden sunlight stored in their bodies through exercise was a psychosomatic treasure to be used as they needed it. That was one of the exercises of *dumo,* or psychic heat, of the Tibetan school of breathing.

It has been known from time immemorial that some people, lightly clad or even naked, possess an extraordinary ability to withstand extreme cold. Travelers in North China, Kashmir, the Himalayas, and Tibet have testified to seeing naked people sitting motionless on the snow or standing in strange attitudes, exposed to wind and freezing temperatures. Near the capital of Kashmir, Shirnigar, hundreds of pilgrims ascend the glacier yearly to reach the Cave of Amar-Natu, to worship there a phallus of ice, sacred to Shiva, Lord of the World. The pilgrims in the procession are completely naked or wear only a loincloth. In the Himalayas and Tibet naked yogis initiated in the art of psychic heat sit cross-legged in bitter cold on the bank of a frozen river or lake. Pieces of cloth of various sizes are dipped into the icy cold water and then draped around the body. At least three pieces of cloth the size of a bedsheet must be dried up in this manner to receive the title *repa*, meaning "cotton-clad." From then on, the yogi wears only light cotton robes even in the severe mountain winter.

In China the tests are more severe. Nine holes are cut in a frozen river and a candidate to shamanship dives into the first hole, swims under the ice to the second, and so on successively to the ninth hole.

This phenomenon is not confined to the East. Initiation by cold is also known to Labrador eskimos. After spending five days and nights in a small kayak in the ocean, one is given the title *angakkok*. In Australia, aborigines are capable of sleeping naked on the bare ground in nearly zero temperatures. In Europe many saints and holy wanderers were known to walk barefoot in the snow, wearing only long cotton gowns.

The art of *dumo (gtum-mo, tummo)* as I am describing it here has its origin in Tibet. Later, it was introduced to India and became an integral part of Kundalini yoga. Before the Chinese invasion of Tibet a number of lama-series offered special courses in developing psychic heat. During complicated and elaborate training, a student learns how to use his powers of concentration, imagination, and willpower, with various breathing techniques as well as meditative practices, to accomplish the goal.

Basically the art of *dumo* is the ability to convert *prana*

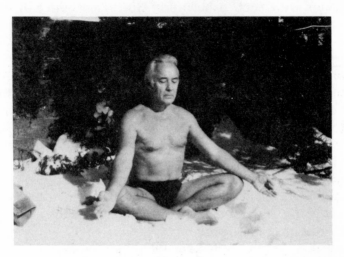

The author practicing *dumo*, Tibetan art of psychic heat, melting the snow.

into the sensation of bodily heat. Training commences with the gradual "toughening" of a student, who is told to dress lightly, spend much time in the open, and never to warm himself by an open fire. From the very first day of training he is told to "think warm," to develop an attitude "I am stronger than cold; I do not fear it."

Exercises are divided into two main groups: internal and external *dumo*. External *dumo* consists of creating a protective aura of warmth around the body, while internal *dumo* involves various techniques of developing heat from within.

Preliminary Exercises

First: Seated cross-legged, rhythmical breath established, the hands are placed on top of each other, palms up. The student is told to imagine a coin resting in the middle of his palm. The coin is getting progressively warmer with each exhalation. After succeeding in this exercise, which largely depends on concentration, hands and feet are warmed in the same manner. The next objective is to warm up the spinal column and then the entire body. In all these exercises, the method is the same. A student visualizes *prana* drawn in with the incoming breath and directed to the focal point in the body with exhalation. He concentrates on converting this energy into the sensation of bodily heat. Success in this exercise varies from person to person. It depends entirely on the power of concentration and on the student's receptivity to autosuggestion. I remember an incident when one of my students sustained an actual burn during the exercise with the imaginary coin.

Second: Another effective technique of *dumo,* which is usually done as a preliminary exercise, consists of deep inhalation and tensing of the entire body. Heat can be developed in a very short time through this technique. For the trained person, only 6 tensings are sufficient to warm up the entire body. Generally speaking, *dumo* is more of a challenge for the mind than for the body. This has also been emphasized by teachers of *dumo,* who suggest that sensations of heat and cold have their origin in the mind.

External Dumo, *or Protective Cocoon*

This is a popular Tibetan exercise of psychic heat. It is also known as the "dress of breath." It could be practiced while sitting, lying down, or walking. With rhythmical breath established, the student imagines that he is directing *prana* through every pore of his skin with each exhalation. He visualizes a protective aura around his body, extending out to a distance of about 4 inches. This cocoon completely surrounds the body. Within it, one feels warm and protected. One concentrates on the mantra *hum* related to the element fire. To be ready to practice this exercise, one must completely conquer the fear of cold. Many weeks of meditative practices precede this exercise so that the unconscious mind is fully conditioned for it.

Internal Dumo, *or Fire Within*

In any traditional cross-legged position, with left nostril closed, the student rapidly breathes through the right nostril, known as the "sun nostril," or "nostril of heat." He concentrates his mind's eye on the *Manipura* chakra, visualizing a tiny flame appearing in this region. When the image is clearly established, he proceeds with breathing through both nostrils, directing *prana* to "feed the flame" and build heat within. He imagines warmth gradually filling his entire body. He is then ready to go out in the bitter cold, warmed up by psychic heat.

Another exercise of internal *dumo* is done on a bright, sunny day. Seated cross-legged in the open, facing the sun, eyes closed, the student covers his left nostril and, lifting his head up, inhales a long breath through the right nostril, imagining that the energy of sunlight is drawn into his body. Inhalation completed, the chin is locked to the chest and the mind concentrated on storing the energy of sunshine in the solar plexus. The energy later can be used in warming up the body as if, by the power of imagination, it were a supply of liquid sunlight stored in the system. Earlier I described the lamas engaged in this exercise.

Cooling Breath

The powers of concentration and imagination play an important part in the following breath controls. Through these powers, cosmic energy in the breath can assume many different forms; *prana* can be transformed into the sensations of heat, cold, or energy. The ability of the student to concentrate makes all the difference in these exercises.

In the context of delaying aging and prolonging the creative part of life, cooling exercises are vitally important. They have to be practiced on a regular basis. Certain techniques eventually must be done not less than 100 times a day on a regular basis. In various treatises of different parts of the East, it is suggested that the life span could be doubled through regular and methodical practice of these exercises. As I have mentioned, one of the modern schools of thought teaches that the span of human life could be doubled if the temperature of the body could be lowered a mere one or two degrees. Scientists don't know how to do it, but *pranayamas* devised possibly 2,000 years ago offer a method. The list of benefits ascribed to these techniques include the extension of life to 150 years and the development of a "luminous body," free from disease and decay.

EXERCISE 1: *Shitali,* or Breath Through Crow's Beak

A number of breathing techniques have been designed from observing the habits, modes of living, and behavior of many animals, birds, and reptiles bestowed with longevity. Tradition says that this breath was designed after observing the manner of breath of a legendary crow who lived hundreds of years. *Jharandasamhita,* another old treatise on yoga, describes the technique as such: "Along the tongue the air is drawn in very slowly until it fills the belly. Hold the breath awhile, breathe out through both nostrils."

In this exercise the tongue is folded lengthwise, a movement that can be achieved readily by some people but which requires an effort by others. The tip of the tongue is protruded about the breadth of the little finger through pursed lips. The air is slowly drawn through the tunnel until the lungs are completely filled. Exhalation is slowly performed through both nostrils. Because the mouth should be kept moist, a tumbler of cold water can be kept nearby to rinse the mouth after every 7 breaths. Twenty-one to 35 breaths are done at one sitting. Traditionally, the exercise should be practiced 3 times a day.

The effect is an increase of physical beauty and prolonged life. *Shivasamhita* claims that this manner of breath also improves eyesight and sense of hearing. It is suggested that the exercise shouldn't be practiced in cold weather. In the tradition of avatara yoga, and if practiced indoors, it can be part of the daily routine throughout the year.

EXERCISE 2: Cold Maker

Closely related to the above exercise, this technique requires that the tongue not be folded but slightly protruded through the lips while the breathing is done the same as above. This is one of the healing breaths of yoga. According to tradition, it cures a number of diseases. It is advisable to practice it during fasting, as it appeases hunger. It also counteracts laziness.

EXERCISE 3: Teeth Breath

In this technique the tip of the tongue touches the soft palate. Breath is inhaled through loosely clenched teeth to make a hissing sound. It is exhaled through the nostrils. In this exercise the mouth is regularly moistened with cold water. The sensation of coolness is developed in the mouth in a short time; eventually, it radiates through the entire body. The exercise lowers body temperature and increases life span.

EXERCISE 4: *Anahata* Breath

Concentration on certain nervous centers of the body produces the sensation of pleasant coolness. A healthy person feels cool around the middle of the chest even during very warm weather. Concentration on the *Anahata* chakra produces a lowering of the body temperature.

In one of the cross-legged poses, the rhythmical breath established, *prana* is directed to the *Anahata* chakra with each exhalation. The mind is concentrated on the pleasant sensation of coolness.

EXERCISE 5: Breath for Cooling the Skin

In this method, *prana* is directed to the skin as if exhalation is occurring not only through the nostrils but through millions of pores of the body. By concentrating, *prana* is converted to the sensation of pleasant coolness.

EXERCISE 6: *Ida* Breath

The left nostril, referred to as *ida,* is the cooling nostril. With eyes closed, inhale and exhale through the left nostril. The mind is concentrated on the sensation of developing pleasant coolness.

EXERCISE 7: *Merudanda* Breath

In this breath the roots of the spinal nerves are points of concentration. It is believed that spinal nerves are greatly susceptible to mental suggestion. After cross-legged pose and rhythmical breath are established, *prana* is sent to the spinal column, with the mind concentrated on the sensation of coolness.

Snake Breath for Skin Rejuvenation

Tradition says that this outstanding breath control was designed by sages of the past after observing the breathing of snakes during their time of changing skins. It is claimed that the snake breath, coupled with certain other techniques and a special diet, lactovegetarian in its essence, can completely rejuvenate the aging skin of the face in six months' time.

Seated in a cross-legged position, one breathes rapidly in and out through the teeth with as much hissing *(sh)* sound as one can produce for half a dozen times, followed by a long inhalation, also through the teeth, and a long exhalation in the same manner. Six cycles of the snake breath are followed by three cycles of the cooling breath, wherein the tip of the tongue touches the palate. Exhalation is done through the nostrils.

This cycle of breathing is completed by "teasing" the soft palate with the tip of the tongue until extensive saliva is produced and swallowed. This cycle should be performed twice a day, morning and evening. Complete treatment includes a watermelon mask in which the face is gently rubbed by a pad of watermelon rind and exposed to the sun until the juice is dried up.

One of my students in Australia, a woman of Dutch-Norwegian descent, at the age of fifty had dried and sun-damaged facial skin. Using this method, she achieved complete rejuvenation of the skin of her face. An extremely dedicated woman, she never missed a single day of her breathing practices, and from the very beginning she had no doubt of her success. That is all it takes to accomplish the rejuvenation.

Chakra Breathing

One of my vivid experiences related to chakras did not occur in a remote ashram of China or India but in a modern hotel in the heart of Chicago only a few years ago. During a convention on yoga meditation and associated practices, I was talking to a man at the end of my address to the public. Suddenly, all lights went off. In complete darkness I saw very clearly a bluish aura surrounding my companion, as well as six circles or chakras of his ethereal body.[11] The image was very vivid. I satisfied myself that those centers indeed exist as a part of man's makeup.

Benefits of chakra breath controls are traditionally described as being on several levels: physical as well as mental and spiritual. In ancient texts there are many suggestions that mental powers can be developed through breath control. The Viassa commentator says, "There is no austerity which leads higher than breath control. It purifies all impurities and the flame of knowledge is kindled." In the tradition of Raja (royal) yoga, there is a belief that nine-tenths of our mental powers are still undeveloped because of lack of correct breathing. There are a number of *pranayamas* dealing with *Brahma* chakra, or upper cortex of the brain, as well as with the six other chakras.

Although many techniques for chakra breathing are esoteric, I have selected a number of breath controls that are suitable for this program. All chakra breath controls are done in the cross-legged position on an empty stomach and while forces of the psyche are in complete balance. The student must feel ready both physically and spiritually, and his mind must be receptive and willing. Chakra breathing enables one to attain a purity so that higher evolvement on the physical, mental, and spiritual planes is possible.

EXERCISE 1: *Muladara* Chakra

The first chakra is located at the base of the spine and is accepted as the seat of Kundalini power, symboli-

11. Another yogic concept teaches the sevenfold composition of man: physical body, ethereal body, astral body, body of mundane thoughts, body of higher thoughts, body of light or soul, and spirit.

cally described as the "sleeping serpent." It is also the seat of excretory energy known as *apana*. With rhythmical breath established, the student forms an image of *prana* directed to this chakra. Concentration on this center leads to physical purity of the body.

EXERCISE 2: *Svadisthana* Breath
The next center is located in the genitals. Directing *prana* to this center leads to control of sexual energy and sexual desire and opens the gates to Kundalini power.

EXERCISE 3: Breath of Energy
The *Manipura* chakra, or solar plexus, is the seat of physical vitality in the body. Many breath controls described previously have this chakra as a point of concentration. With deep and rhythmical breathing established, the mind is concentrated on the thought of *prana* separated from the breath and stored in this center.

EXERCISE 4: Breath of *Anahata* Chakra
This *pranayama* involves concentrating on the middle of the chest, or the cardiac plexus, while breathing slowly and rhythmically. This breath control plays a very important part in promoting longevity. The basic thought behind this exercise is the stimulation of the cardiac plexus and slowing down the biological clock. The mind is also concentrated on the thought of longevity.

EXERCISE 5: *Vishuddha* Chakra
This chakra corresponds to the part of the neck where four important endocrine glands are located: thyroid, parathyroid, salivary, and adenoid. Those glands, considered very important in physical yoga, play an important part in a physiological balance of the body. With rhythmical breath established, concentration is on directing *prana* to this center.

EXERCISE 6: Concentration Between Eyebrows

Breath is directed to the point between the eyebrows known as the "third eye," or *Ajna* chakra, the seat of higher faculties of man as well as the center of enlightenment. The length of the exercise is individually determined. Usually, not less than half an hour is devoted to this breathing meditation.

EXERCISE 7: Purification of the Mind

With rhythmical breath established, the student forms an image of *prana* directed to the head, purifying his mind from all negative, low, or sad thoughts. Graphically, it is expressed as a dark cloud gradually forced off the mind and floating away, while underneath the cloud is a vision of pure light. This exercise is an actual effort of the will to reprogram the mind and to move onto a higher plane of consciousness.

Healing Breathing

One's inner confidence to deal with illness is directly related to longevity. The history of healing breathing is as old as mankind. It was mentioned in *The Egyptian Book of the Dead,* in ancient Chinese treatises, as well as in the traditional Indian literature. Teachings present a remarkable claim that any disease can be either cured or arrested by breathing exercises, diet, and a mental state of peace. In modern China, not less than thirty clinics are in operation, using the principles of a remarkable healing breath known as *chigoon*. Its main doctrine teaches that cosmic energy in the air, called *chi*, can be controlled through breathing, accumulating in the body an increased power of resistance to disease. It can also be directed by breath to the seat of the malady with a healing effect. Restoration of the flow of *chi* through the main channels of the body leads to complete recovery. In its basic principle it is close to the ideas of acupuncture. Instead of the actual needle, a needle of concentrated thought or a beam of life force is used to restore the flow of vital energy. Spectacular recoveries have been reported in cases where orthodox medicine has failed.

It is also interesting to note that in the 1950s principles of *chigoon* were introduced in Russia, where it became a very popular method of treatment known there as "pneumotherapy." Multitudes of various maladies, from emphysema of the lungs to schizophrenia are treated in Russia and China by this method.

In the context of prolonging life and staying healthy, healing breath is indispensable. It is an additional and powerful tool to fight the ravages of time. Knowledge of it adds to the inner strength of the practicer, which is a very important factor in gaining mastery over the passage of time.

Five Manners of Healing Breath

One of the unusual aspects of the Chinese school of breathing is a claim that a man can breathe in five different ways: He can make the breath hug the left inner walls of both nostrils, or the right inner walls, or the top inner walls, or the lower inner walls. The fifth way of breathing is our normal breathing, in which breath goes through the middle of the nostrils. This claim most likely will startle and surprise the orthodox trained medical doctor who may dismiss the whole theory as utter nonsense. Yet it survived in the East for hundreds of years and was successfully used by countless numbers of people seeking health by breath control. A possible biological explanation of this phenomenon is that our nostrils contain many nervous fibers which branch into the cortex of the brain. Through concentration, we can learn how to influence the direction of this energy to afflicted parts of the body.

The benefits attached to the five manners of breathing are as follows: Making the breath hug the left inner walls of the nostrils is beneficial to the heart, while direct breathing to the right side of the nostrils is beneficial to the lungs and chest; direct breathing to the lower inner part of the nostrils is beneficial to the stomach and urinary system, and direct breathing along the upper walls of the nostrils is beneficial in cases of mental afflictions, including psychosomatic ones; normal breathing, directed through the middle of the nostrils, is suggested for relaxation and various meditative practices. In addition, it is taught that we can make the right or left nostril the dominant one by an effort of concentration, and thereby control even more the beneficial effects of our breathing.

In *chigoon* the physiology of breath is closely associated with metaphysics. Concentration always plays a most important role. Beneficial results can't be achieved without concentration.

Chigoon is mainly a method of self-healing through breath, but the trained practitioner can become a healer. In this case a basic principle is the transfer of life force from healer to patient. It is done either by direct control (laying on of the hands with gentle pressure) or purely by mental concentration. *Chi* can be directed to a mental image of the sick person, irrespective of the distance separating the healer from the subject. The one who desires to be a healer must learn how to build his own life force by breathing exercises and should always be cautious not to drain himself completely in the process of helping others. Otherwise he can fall an easy prey to many diseases.

In a book of this size it is impossible to give complete

coverage of all the healing techniques of Chinese, Indian, and Tibetan breath controls, but I will present a selection of the most important methods in the context of healing. The following are heart healing breaths, based on physiology and supported by metaphysics.

The main principle of the heart healing breaths is the emphasis on exhalation, retention of emptiness, and undoubted belief in ultimate success. The power of the imagination also plays a very important role. The practicer trains his mind to visualize an actual expansion of cardiovascular arteries with each outgoing breath.

Healing Breath for Angina

EXERCISE 1

This exercise usually is done in a sitting position but also can be done lying on the back. After rhythmical breath is established and the body is completely relaxed, a mental image of the heart and cardiovascular system is brought into the mind. Physiology teaches us that during exhalation the /arteries of the cardiovascular system are expanded. One concentrates on an image of the arteries expanding during exhalation. Duration of this exercise is usually 5–15 minutes.

EXERCISE 2

Assume a cross-legged position. The left arm is raised to symbolize an antenna for receiving *prana* while the right hand, with the fist closed, is placed across the chest and against the heart. During deep inhalation, the mind is concentrated on *prana* drawn from the air and directed to the heart. With exhalation, the left arm is brought down and into contact with the right fist, which in turn produces an actual massaging effect on the heart. The breath is completely exhaled and emptiness is retained for a few seconds. The left arm is raised again. The procedure is repeated 12 times.

EXERCISE 3

Seat yourself in a cross-legged position, with the left hand grasping the right wrist and placed on top of the head. After a full inhalation, both arms are raised straight up, effecting a squeezing pressure on both sides of the chest. Breath and position are retained for 4 heartbeats. Then the arms are lowered to the original position while breath is exhaled.

EXERCISE 4

Same as above, but instead of placing the arms on top of the head, place them in the middle of the chest (in the same attitude). When breath is inhaled, both arms are stretched forward away from the body, creating pressure on the sides of the chest. Six repetitions.

EXERCISE 5

Seat yourself in a cross-legged position, close the right nostril with the thumb, and take a slow breath through the left nostril, each time emphasizing exhalation.

EXERCISE 6

Take a supine position, place fingertips lightly in the middle of the chest, establish a rhythmical breath, and concentrate the mind on an image of the life force directed to the cardiac plexus with a stimulating effect.

EXERCISE 7

Seated in a cross-legged position, breathe through both nostrils, with the breath hugging the left inner side of the nostrils and the mind concentrated on the powerful healing effects of this breath.

All-Healing Breath

The ancient belief that a certain amount of life force flows out from the fingertips with each exhalation, forming fields of energy, has been recently verified by science.

There are three main techniques wherein *prana* is directed back into the system with healing and energizing effects.

1. Seated on the floor, stretch legs forward while index fingers are locked against the big toes. In this attitude, deep and rhythmical breath is established and an image of the life force circulating round and round in the system is formed.

2. As above. Legs are brought over the head toward the floor behind while the hands are stretched over the head to hold the toes with the feet apart.

3. Angular stretching pose (see illustration, p. 150).

In all these three poses, the life force is locked into the system. A toning and invigorating effect is experienced by every vital organ of the body.

Breathing Away the Malady

This is one of the basic exercises in the tradition of all yogas. In the supine position, deep and rhythmical breath established, the mind is concentrated on the thought that, with each exhalation, cosmic energy is directed through thousands of pores of the body, forcing the malady out of the system.

In the practices of Chinese healing breath controls, diseases are divided into three categories: light, mild, and severe. The healing principles of the severe maladies include very carefully selected light diet, peaceful rural surroundings, and breathing three times a day in four different positions: fifteen minutes while sitting in a chair; or cross-legged fifteen minutes while lying on the right side; fifteen minutes while lying on the left side; and fifteen minutes while lying on the back. Altogether, there is one hour for each session in the morning, one in the afternoon, and one in the evening. For three hours daily the patient breathes in these postures in a completely relaxed attitude. He is for three hours a day in a self-induced "alpha" state of consciousness most conducive to healing.

Breath to Create Fields of Energy

Outstanding among healing breaths is the cycle of techniques combining ideas of Yantra yoga with concentrated breathing. Yantra yoga is described as the "yoga of geometric forms," and in this practice invisible fields of energy are created within the human body. Apart from rhythmical breathing which is combined with all the exercises, these methods, in my opinion, are of purely psychosomatic origin. Outstanding among these practices is the creation of the imaginary hexagram in the human body which, later on, is used as the basis for concentration and contemplation.

EXERCISE 1: *Yantra* Breath
    In the pose of an adept, with the back and neck in a straight line, hands resting on the knees in the *mudra of knowledge,* a point in the left shoulder is activated by breath. The next breath is directed to the right shoulder, and the third breath is directed to the base of the spine. The practicer is told to imagine a triangle appearing in his body. The fourth breath is directed to the right knee, the fifth to the left knee, and the sixth to a point between the eyebrows, forming the second triangle. Now

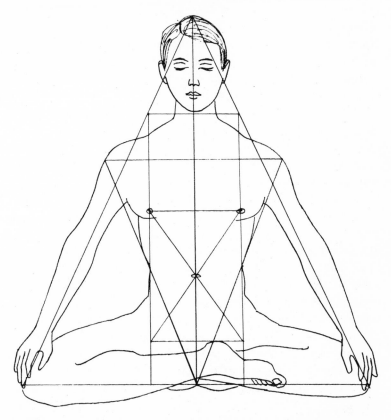

Fields of energy in the human body, according to Chinese tradition. (*Drawing by Daphne Hewson*)

two interlocked triangles are visualized by the practicer, one having its apex in the *Muladara* chakra, the other in the *Ajna* chakra. The practicer concentrates on the image of two interlocked triangles drawn by the power of imagery into his body. The hexagram, commonly known as the Star of David, has a much longer tradition. It was known as an early Sumerian symbol of the world— three points in space (length, width, and breadth) and three points in time (past, present, and future). By describing this symbol upon his body, the practicer unites himself with universal principles. Holding in his mind this *yantra,* he breathes deeply and rhythmically for not less than 15 minutes. This technique has a remarkably energizing effect on the entire body and is credited with curing many diseases, as well as delaying aging processes in the body.

EXERCISE 2: Slowing the Time Clock

This method is even more involved than the previous one. Seated as before, the left arm is raised straight over the head while the right hand touches the ground. Both hands are locked in the *mudra of knowledge.* Rhythmical breath is established. The practicer imagines that he draws *prana* through the air with his left hand, forming a channel going across his chest and into the right arm and into the earth. After half a dozen breaths in this attitude, when the clear image of the channel is established, the arms change positions and the right hand is raised in the air while the left hand touches the ground. An image of the second channel crossing the first is established. The same number of breaths are performed. Both arms are raised now, forming an image of a point of energy created in the middle of the cardiac *(Anahata)* chakra. The practicer breathes until he experiences tiredness in both arms, with the mind concentrated on the thought of slowing the inner time pace in his cardiac plexus.

EXERCISE 3: Curing the Headache
There are three main techniques for curing a headache.

First, on one's back, with rhythmical breath established, concentrate on the big toes. When complete concentration is accomplished, the headache is cured.

Second, in the sitting position, bring the fingertips together, concentrating upon developing heat in the fingertips. When the sensation of warmth is developed, the headache is usually gone. The technique is now used successfully at the Menninger Clinic to cure migraine headaches.

A *third* technique involves creating a field of energy in the head. The first breath is directed through the right ear, the second through the left ear, while the third is through the top of the head. When the image of the triangle is established, practice breathing rhythmically, concentrating simultaneously on these three points. With each exhalation, breathe the headache away through the three points of *yantra.*

EXERCISE 4: Afflictions of the Chest and Stomach
These afflictions are treated by creating the chest *yantra.* First, breath is directed to the right nipple, second to the left, and third to the navel. Concentration is on a powerful field of energy and the sensation of warmth which helps to overcome whatever disorder is in question.

EXERCISE 5: Disorders of the Urinary Tract
These disorders are treated by the triangle created by directing the breath to the left groin, right groin, and

navel. Concentration on these two *yantras* combined is a powerful creator of a point of pulsating energy in the navel.

Analyzing the methods described, one could conclude that they are perhaps exercises developing constructive thinking. Everything that starts in the mind can be erased by mental effort. In the context of "age unlimited," these unusual techniques of self-healing should not be discarded lightly. An inner knowledge of self-healing powers gives the student additional strength to fight the passage of time and eventually to achieve mastery over it.

Time and Breath

Some years ago I was conducting a class in a big, well-appointed private home. As I was discussing various breath controls with a group of students, I was conscious of the continuous ticking of the big grandfather clock behind me in the hall. Suddenly, I was made aware again of something I learned much earlier in my life: that this uniform ticking of the clock was not the same for everyone in the room, that each creature on this earth has his or her own time pace, or biological clock, which moves at its own unique speed.

As an extreme example of a tragically rapid biological clock, we might consider the mysterious and dreadful disease known as progeria, which can cause a child to die of old age. In progeria, the biological clock is running so incredibly fast that the aging processes are speeded up to at least ten times the normal rate. A child of perhaps seven years of age who suffers from this disease will die gray-headed and toothless, its face full of wrinkles and its inner organs and blood vessels as worn as though it were a hundred years old.

On the other hand, if the aging process can run haywire

one way, madly accelerating its pace, then it is only logical to assume that the contrary is also possible. One of the greatest attainments of an adept in either of the three yogas is "mastery over passing time," or, in other words, the ability at will to slow down the biological clock so that the life span is greatly extended. India, Tibet, and China are full of legends of great masters who are said to be 500 or 600 years old. Incredible as that sounds, modern scientists also believe that, at least theoretically, such an extension of the individual life is possible. To achieve such longevity would, of course, require ideal environmental conditions and a perfectly balanced diet. Science admits that the ideal diet (that is, a diet that would permit a more or less perfect balance between the death rate and birth rate of body cells) is not yet known.

In China, I learned some meditative practices directed toward recognition of the time pace within. We will return to this subject in chapter 13 on meditation, but here I would like to mention that awareness of one's internal clock leads gradually to control over its pace. The secret of controlling the biological clock is contained in the art and science of breathing. When breathing is slowed down, the biological clock is also slowed down.

Further, during the deep, dreamless sleep of the first state of unconsciousness, time literally stands still for us. The fact that we do not age nearly so fast during sleep has led to the suggestion by modern gerontologists that people could live to age 150 if only they could be taught to hibernate. Of course, hibernation is a rather dull method of prolonging the life span. We are here to live and enjoy fully the great adventure of life, which is hardly synonymous with hibernation. Yoga offers a much more sophisticated method of achieving the same results in its exercises that are based on an awareness of the connection between the march of time and the manner of breathing.

Anyone who learns to slow the rhythm of his breathing will slow the speed with which his biological clock measures out his life span. Slowing down the rate of breathing affects the upper cortex of the brain, slows the pulse and lowers the blood pressure, and results in a mental state of tranquility, which is so important in prolonging the life span.

6

Energy from the Elements

All rivers are flowing through my veins. All clouds are reflected in my eyes. All mountains are locked in my body. I am earth, air, I am everything.

—Chinese poet

Everyone who has had the experience of escaping from a long, bleak, northern winter into the warm sunshine, blue waters, and golden sun of a southern climate will agree that two weeks of complete relaxation on a Pacific or Caribbean seashore will do more for your sense of well-being than any known medicine. Instinctively we seek rejuvenation from the elements when we go on vacations. For centuries, yogis have included this intimate contact with earth, air, water, and sunshine as an important part of their regimen.

My Chinese master at the ashram in the South Sea who specialized in rejuvenation was, in his own way, a dedicated and serious scientist as well as a yogi. He accepted into his ashram people over age sixty-five and worked with them for nine months, a period symbolic of gestation. In preparing for the "new birth" of his students, his chief "attendants" were sunshine, the beautiful air of his ashram, the unpolluted water of the sea surrounding the island, and the virgin golden sand of the island's small lagoon. His only "medicines" were breathing exercises and gymnastics performed thrice a day.

Everyone was compelled to get up with the sunrise, and by sunset the little oil lamps in the rooms had to be extinguished. Food in his ashram was simple and wholesome, sustaining and well balanced. It included vegetables, some fruits and berries, soybean milk, and soybean curd. Great emphasis was placed on purification of the body. On meeting the new students, the master always examined their tongues and the retinas of their eyes. In almost all cases the newcomers had to endure three days of fasting, aided by the tea of purgative herbs.

Each day started with meditative practices, breathing exercises, and an hour of Taoist yoga, followed by a simple breakfast and two hours of rest. At midmorning, an hour's set of exercises focused on harboring the energies of sunlight, water, air, and earth. This set was repeated early in the evening, followed by more breath controls and other exercises. A half hour of meditation ended the day.

This program—meditation, breath control, diet, and techniques to absorb energies from the elements—resulted in some cases of rejuvenation that I observed personally and can only describe as astounding. People regained their suppleness, muscle tone, and healthy skin. All their bodily functions were greatly improved. During these nine months, some people became twenty years younger.

The main doctrine of this master was that uniting one's body with the surrounding elements could recharge the body with energy and restore it to perfect balance and health. Included below are exercises related to each of the four elements I have mentioned. The element of fire is represented by the energy of sunlight.

As a matter of interest, the element of fire is used for purifying and recharging by some metaphysical schools in China as well as in India. Although I do not recommend these practices for the Westerner, I would like to describe briefly some of the esoteric ceremonies involving the element of fire before proceeding with the exercises recommended for the student. Certain initiation ceremonies involve the adept sitting surrounded by four camp fires with the fifth fire—the midday sun—above his head. Fire walking is also a part of initiation ceremonies practiced even today in various parts of the world. The remarkable thing about fire walking is that often, inspired by the master, onlookers follow him through the long pit of red hot coals without any ill effects.

One of the ceremonies I observed in South China was done in such a manner: Early in the morning a trench about twenty feet long and three feet wide was dug and filled with firewood that had been liberally splashed with kerosene and oil. When this was lighted, the ditch was transformed into a roaring inferno. By midday, after the fire had burned for two or three hours, there were red-hot coals with tongues of bluish flame where the fire had been.

At a prearranged time, the barefooted master, dressed only in a small loincloth, appeared from his quarters. Walking to the edge of the pit, he put his big toe among the coals in a gesture like that of a cautious swimmer trying the temperature of the water before plunging. He then proclaimed the fire not hot enough for purification! With muffled exclamations of amazement and delight, his disciples and some onlookers rushed to the pit, waving large palm branches to fan the flames. In a short while the fire was a mass of fiercely glowing red charcoal. The master nodded his head in satisfaction. For a moment he stood at the edge of the pit, feet together, palms pressed in the attitude of prayer. He then stepped right into the mass of red charcoal and crossed the pit with deliberately slow strides. A few of his disciples followed, as well as a number of onlookers. Afterward, none showed any signs of being burned.

I asked the master how he was able to do it. He sat in silence for quite some time before he told me, "I really don't know how I did it. But prior to my walk I meditated for two hours, gradually working myself into a state of unquestioned belief that I would not be hurt. That is, I suppose, the secret." He offered the explanation that those who followed him were moved by his example, which triggered the same faith deep in their psyches.

Without going so far as to walk on fire, there are many things we can do to nurture ourselves with the energies of the elements. The pleasures of nature—sunbathing, swimming, fresh air, soft grass, and sand—are known to everyone. By becoming conscious of our great need to remain in close, constant contact with the elements, we might do much to improve our health and increase our vitality through this medium. For instance, it is important to gather as much winter sunshine into the body as we can manage even if we have to do our "sunning" while partially clothed. We can use our minds to lead us consciously into other "recharging" experiences. Below are some suggestions to begin with.

Energy from the Sunlight

In all exercises involving the sun, wise discretion should be used to determine the amount of time that you, individually, can spend in the sun without harm. People's ability to tolerate sunlight varies. Be aware of your own.

EXERCISE 1

In the inner courtyard of the ashram described above was an ancient circular stone, large and heavy, covered by half-worn characters in what looked like the Chinese zodiac signs. The stone was pivoted on another stone so precisely that it could be turned around with little difficulty. My teacher once remarked that when his ashram was built hundreds of years ago, the stone was already there. The ashram literally was built around it. He said that he tried to estimate the age of the stone but could not, even approximately, because most of the inscription was worn out by the passage of time. He suggested that in all probability it dated to Chinese prehistory and was a relic of the sun worshipers who once dwelt upon the island. We called it the "sun stone." An unforgettable experience was to take a sunbath while sitting on the stone.

The exercise was practiced by two students during the morning when the sun was not very strong. One student sat in the cross-legged position on the stone while the other slowly turned the stone clockwise until a complete revolution was achieved in a prearranged span of time, usually half an hour. The sunbather wore only a small triangle of loincloth and seated himself on a piece of felt covered by linen. With eyes closed, he began in a position facing the sun to practice deep and rhythmical breathing. He concentrated fully on the thought that with each inhalation he was absorbing the energy of the sunlight into every pore of his skin and with each exhalation he was transforming it into personal energy. We had been instructed by the teacher that the secret of success is concentration, one-pointedness of the mind. In the course of the exercise, while completing a full revolution, every part of one's body was exposed to the sunlight. One finished the exercise by facing the sun again. When the exercise was finished, the students usually changed positions, and the one who had the sunbath then turned the stone for his friend. In this fashion the pleasures of breathing beautiful and pure morning air and feeling the gentle warming touch of sunlight were accentuated by the deep mystical sensation of contact with this ancient stone.

Of course, this exercise can be done without the sun stone, since there is only one in the world of the sort I have described. Everything else can be done as prescribed, with the student turning his body clockwise every few minutes by his own effort until a complete revolution is accomplished and he faces the sun where he began.

EXERCISE 2

This exercise is for the eyesight. Facing the sun in a cross-legged position with eyes closed, move the head slowly from side to side, bathing the closed eyes in the rays of sunlight until the first tears appear. Breath is deep and rhythmical.

EXERCISE 3

The seven chakras of the body can be energized by the sun if one exposes each chakra to the sun for the duration (at first) of 3 slow breaths. Facing the sun as before, with chin pressed to chest, the *Brahma* chakra at the top of the head is exposed to the sun first. Next, the head is raised upward and the mind concentrated on the point between the eyebrows, or the *Ajna* chakra. Then the body is leaned backward and supported with the hands. The chin is raised, exposing the neck region of the thyroid and parathyroid glands (*Vishuddha* chakra) to the sun. The fourth point of concentration is the *Anahata* chakra, by which we energize the cardiac plexus. Then we focus energy onto the solar plexus

(*Manipura* chakra), the genital organs (*Svadisthana* chakra), and finally the base of the spine (*Muladara* chakra).

During all these practices, a student is advised to concentrate on the thought that he is actually drawing the energy of sunlight through each of the psychic centers with a stimulating and energizing effect. Starting with only 3 breaths, the number of breaths dedicated to each chakra is then raised to 7 and eventually to 21.

EXERCISE 4

Throat Exercise

A very popular exercise, this one can be practiced daily when the weather permits. Sunning of the throat is done first while seated in a cross-legged position facing the sun, with eyes closed. The mouth is opened wide while the tongue is protruded, admitting sunshine as deeply into the throat as possible.

Dog's Breath

With the mouth wide open and tongue out, vigorous breaths can be inhaled and exhaled through the mouth in very much the same way as a dog pants. Duration: 6 breaths.

Only 3 rounds of each technique should be done at one sitting.

Energy from the Earth

EXERCISE 1: Embracing Mother Earth

At the ashram, one of the very few exercises in which everyone participated together instead of working individually was charging the body with the energy of Mother Earth. It consists of lying on warm sand or ground, breathing deeply, first on the back, then on the right side and the left, as well as flat on the stomach with the arms alongside the body. Concentrate on absorbing energy from the earth. The exercise should last 15–20 minutes.

EXERCISE 2: Touching for Energy

Another technique is performed in the cross-legged sitting position with hands in the *mudra of knowledge* position (see p. 81), pointed down so that fingertips make contact with the earth. The student forms an image of the energy of Mother Earth drawn in with inhalation and transformed to personal energy with exhalation.

EXERCISE 3: Smell of Good Earth

The next exercise consists of turning up some earth, building a small mound of it, bringing the face close to the mound, supporting the body with the hands, and establishing rhythmical breathing for 2–3 minutes. The thought is the same as in the previous exercise: With incoming breath, energy from the earth is transferred into personal energy. The wholesome, potent smell of the earth enhances the exercise.

Energy from the Air

EXERCISE 1: Air Bath

This exercise is one of the most loved and commonly performed exercises of the student of breath control. It can be done either in a cross-legged position or lying supine. With rhythmical breath established, the mind is concentrated on the thought that the entire body is breathing. One is inhaling and exhaling through millions of pores of the skin, with *prana* penetrating every cell of the body. Breathing in this manner eventually leads to the sensation of merging with the air, a feeling of transparency or bodilessness, as in yoga *nidra* (see p. 72). The exercise always has a beautiful recharging effect if done with full concentration.

EXERCISE 2: Pranic Antennae

Seated cross-legged with both arms raised above the head, palms facing each other at about the width of the shoulders, spread the fingers to form antennae. Establish rhythmical breath. The student forms an image of the life force drawn through the fingertips into his system with inhalation and transformed into his own energy with exhalation. One continues the exercise until there is a slight sensation of tiredness in the raised arms.

EXERCISE 3: Pose of the Frog *(Manduka Asana)*

Seated as above, the palms are raised up and placed together just above the crown of the head. Again, the fingers play the role of antennae or points of concentration, absorbing *prana* with incoming breath and trans-- forming it into personal energy with outgoing breath. A variation of the same exercise is done while sitting on the back of the heels with knees one foot apart, arms and palms in the same position as above. This posture promotes full abdominal breathing and is often used as an exercise to perfect the full abdominal breath.

Energy from the Water

It is taught both in Oriental and Occidental philosophies that life started in the primordial ocean. That is why unification with the water, especially the water of the ocean, is so beautifully refreshing.

EXERCISE 1: Contact with the Water

Every time you take a swim, a shower, or even a simple wash, you are recharging your vitality by the energy of the water. An important aspect of morning purification is a bath, or at least sponging your body with a cloth.

EXERCISE 2: Floating Fish

A classical exercise of recharging oneself by the element of water is to float in the water in the posture of a fish with legs locked in the lotus position, arms (with fingers interlaced) under the neck. Anyone who is capable of locking legs in this position will be amazed how easy it is to float in this attitude. The orthodox floating on the back with the legs straight could be practiced if the lotus position has not been mastered. As in all exercises involving the elements, one absorbs *prana* with incoming breath and transforms it into personal energy with outgoing breath.

7

Diet and Fasting

We are what we eat.
—Proverb

Any program for health and longevity should give early attention to diet because it is so important an influence on our physical condition and our frame of mind. The subject of diet has received an enormous amount of attention recently, so much so that it would seem we are in the midst of a diet revolution. That possibility could be seen as good news were it not for the fact that no one is certain where the revolution will take us in terms of health. Perhaps I should say that there is too much certainty among too many diverse points of view. It can be asserted safely, I think, that a diet has not yet been discovered that will serve the needs of everyone.

Our current controversy over diet has a longer history than we might suppose. Over a period of about fifty years I have attended at least 100 diet conferences throughout the world. I have heard vegetarians venomously confronting meat eaters and meat eaters denouncing vegetarians, as well as people who believe in the virtues of one food above all others. The points of view at these conferences often reached extremes of absurdity. For instance, at one

125

conference in Australia, an advocate of eggs presented a hard-boiled egg to every person in the audience, with the suggestion that the egg symbolizes new life and should be ingested as such. Another gentleman passed out raw eggs, and to make a dramatic point—that eggs were good only to be destroyed—invited the audience to throw the eggs at him, which they obligingly did.

Anyone attending these conferences was much more likely to become confused than enlightened on the subject of diet. Nevertheless, there are some guidelines that can be drawn from a study of the effects of different diets on human health and longevity.

Diet habits throughout the world have evolved largely on the basis of climate and resources. One cannot expect an Eskimo to be a vegetarian, given the conditions of his environment. Eastern Indians cannot, as a matter of ecology, cultivate the habit of beef eating when a cow will feed so many more people alive than when slaughtered. Perhaps our own growing awareness of ecology will turn more of us to vegetarianism. Meanwhile, I think most of us are creatures of ethnic habit: We are satisfied best when eating the kinds of foods our ancestors ate.

In countries where food resources are limited, selection in diet is not so great a problem as in affluent countries where foods of all descriptions are available in abundance. In Europe and America, both "middle regions" between extremely hot and extremely cold climates, we have developed the habit of eating a variety of foods from the vegetable, fruit, and meat categories. Over centuries we have evolved complicated cuisines that make it difficult for us to think in terms of simple hunger. Yet that is precisely where our program for rejuvenation through diet should begin: We need to think reflectively about our diet habits and to revise them as necessary to promote health and long life.

The traditional yoga diet is basically lactovegetarian—that is, a combination of vegetables, fruits, and milk products. It is designed to satisfy a sense of healthy hunger. I am aware that it may not be wise to advocate a predominantly vegetarian diet to Westerners who have long-established habits of eating meat. My purpose is not to convert but to encourage thoughtfulness and the development of healthy choice. I should like to begin by describing a program of diet followed in one ashram where I spent some time. You will be able to decide whether the program can be modified to suit your personal needs.

In the yogic tradition, prior to the beginning of physical training, an entire week is dedicated to purification of the body. This week of purification eventually becomes a seasonal pattern of the yoga pupil, practiced in winter, spring, summer, and autumn. The spring purification is considered the most important, since it is believed that in the spring the forces of nature support the practicer. Everything is passing through the cycle of rejuvenation in the spring, and "the wise yogi who steps into this cycle" can be rejuvenated as well.

Traditionally, the week of purification is carried out in the following manner: The first twenty-four hours involves a complete abstention from food (only water is consumed). The next day, the fast is broken by adding fruit or vegetable juice, followed by a solid fruit of one kind (apple, pear, banana, grapes). On the remaining days of the week, four foods are taken: fruits, vegetables, nuts, honey. They are eaten raw or lightly cooked, in moderation, and they are thoroughly chewed.

In the ashram which specialized in rejuvenation, food was rationed. In the beginning it was extremely difficult to be satisfied with the amount of food served. The master told us again and again that we could be satisfied. He wouldn't give us any more food but encouraged us to take longer to eat the food we had been served. He suggested chewing every morsel about twenty times, counting as we chewed, learning to savor every mouthful. "Remember," he often added, gravely shaking his head, "that millions of people in this world are starving." Those who followed him soon learned to be completely satisfied on very small amounts of food. His eating habits involved a periodic modified fast during which he slowly and deliberately chewed half a dozen walnuts and a handful of raisins each midday. He considered that sufficient fuel from one day to the next, at least on a periodic basis. On several occasions I experimented with his diet and found him right.

Eating a meal in the ashram was a form of elaborate meditation. Food was always eaten slowly, thoroughly, and in silence. We were never allowed to drink any water with meals, with the admonition that to do so would dilute stomach juices and upset digestion. Strangely, the joy of eating food in this manner is not lesser but greater than the joy of eating in the conventional way when the mind is preoccupied with something else.

The people who came to the ashram with weight problems were trained to meditate on weight loss. They were encouraged to "think thin" throughout their waking moments. The weight losses were astonishing. Later, introducing this principle of thinking thin to my own students, I noticed that on many occasions they were able to lose weight without changing diets, as if the power of the mind could induce some biochemical change in the body.

Today, I am convinced that it is not what we eat that matters so much as how we eat and how much. Most Westerners, particularly Americans, eat far too much and without respect to proper mastication. We gulp our food while our minds are elsewhere, thus missing whatever pleasure there may be in eating the rich food we so like to anticipate.

In the Western world, overeating has become a way of life. From early childhood, health is equated with the ability to eat prodigious amounts of food. Mothers are proud of their children for eating enormous breakfasts, snacking throughout the day, and consuming a full adult meal in the evening. Furthermore, at one diet conference I attended, a doctor proclaimed that in America an adult leading a sedentary life might eat as much as four times what healthy hunger would require. In my opinion, overeating is one of the major problems of the affluent Western world.

Those who are interested in rejuvenation or in prolonging a healthy life should give serious consideration to eating habits, with special attention to food selection, the amount consumed, and proper digestion, which begins with mastication. Below are some of the guidelines that might be followed.

One generalization we can make safely, I think, is that natural foods—that is, foods that have not been contaminated with chemicals—are more wholesome than commercially prepared foods. That is one sphere in which consciousness raising has had some impressive results, especially in America where packaged produce had replaced almost entirely the more wholesome homegrown foods that were the norm until the past several decades. The "health food" market has grown considerably in the past ten years. Although denounced by adversaries as extravagant in their claims, advocates of health foods such as organically grown vegetables and fruits, wholegrain breads and cereals, nuts, and honey have made an impact on the commercial food market. Aware of the growing demand for uncontaminated produce, many commercial food distributors are following the health food trend by proclaiming on their packages that certain of their foods contain only natural ingredients. This concession has made it possible for the consumer to be more selective about food quality, even when unable to join the growing number of people who grow their own vegetables in home gardens.

Besides avoiding foods containing chemical additives, one should take care whenever possible to choose fresh rather than frozen, packaged, or canned products. The technology of food preservation adversely affects the quality of food; in such a way, paradoxically, the rising standard of life diminishes the pleasure of living. My refrigerator stays relatively empty most of the time because I like to shop daily for what I will eat that day or the next. This shopping pattern may be troublesome to some, but if time permits, it is a much more satisfying way to shop than on a weekly or biweekly basis. Regardless of the convenience of frozen and packaged foods, I believe some important nutritional value is lost in storing food, not to mention deterioration in taste and appearance.

There are a few foods that I recommend avoiding altogether, such as animal fats, refined sugar, flour, and cereals. If you love sweets, honey or brown sugar can be enjoyed instead of refined sugar. Wholegrain cereals and flour are generally available now. Fats may not be exceedingly harmful (a controversial subject), but they are very treacherous to the diet because they contain so many calories. One can be perfectly healthy without eating butter or heavy cream and especially animal fats. A balanced diet will give the body its required amount of fat from meat or milk or nuts.

That brings us to eating habits. The golden rule of diet is never to overeat. You can train yourself to distinguish healthy hunger from false appetite. If you eliminate white bread, cereals, and sugar from your diet, you will eliminate some of the cravings of false appetite. Carbohydrates in general tend to increase one's sense of false hunger; shortly after eating them, one feels hungry again. With protein, the appetite is satisfied longer. Even protein can be overingested, however. Obviously, a marathon runner or a weight lifter needs an abundance of protein. If you are past middle age or if your life is mainly sedentary, you should take proteins in moderate amounts. Bread also needs to be taken moderately because of its high caloric content.

One effective way to measure hunger is to avoid eating when you first get up in the morning and to avoid giving in to the first "gnawings" of appetite that may appear about midmorning. You may be surprised to find that this apparent hunger will disappear soon after it manifests itself. See how long you can go without actually feeling weak. Then eat a banana and measure again how long it is before you feel hunger. Most people find they do want to eat a meal near midday, and that is perhaps the best time to eat—sometime between noon and sunset. For those who find they do need breakfast, a light one is recommended. The same is true for those who need to eat late in the day. In the evening, one can drink a glass of warm water with honey and lemon. That will satisfy hunger and aid digestion as well. Eating only when you are hungry will help you to maintain correct weight; according to many centenarians, it is one of the secrets of their long lives.

For efficient digestion, one should include plenty of vitamins and roughage. A variety of vegetables and fruits will provide both, especially if supplemented with portions of yogurt and honey. The latter are considered "miracle" foods by many current researchers into diet. They have been staples of yogic diet for centuries. Honey contains a variety of vitamins which are badly needed by the system and which are robbed from grains when they are refined. It is widely used to prevent and cure arthritis (recipe: a large spoon of natural honey and a few drops of lemon juice taken each morning in a tumbler of hot water). Yogurt is widely recognized now for its beneficial effects on health. It consists of a very powerful sour milk bacillus which, when introduced into the intestines, can be compared to a friendly army fighting all sorts of harmful bacteria as it "cleans" the intestines. One theory says that aging is partially caused by poisonous bacilli in the intestines which eventually reach every cell of the body.

Yogurt is an effective internal cleanser for the intestines, in addition to being nutritious. Other natural laxatives include fruits known as "brooms of nature"—pears (to be taken on an empty stomach), plums and figs (for after dinner). Watermelon can be taken to cleanse the urinary system. These fruits should be eaten for two to three days or until they complete their cleansing work.

A point should be made about vitamin supplements. As one grows older and the balance of health becomes more unpredictable, vitamin supplements can provide a kind of insurance that one's diet is adequate. Most gerontologists suggest that people after fifty should have a regular intake of vitamins A, B, C, D, and E. They also suggest that vitamin C should be taken along with other vitamins to help the system absorb them. Some suggest that a daily dose of 400 units of vitamin E and 1,000 units of vitamin C is an adequate supplement. You can always consult your family physician for an assessment of your particular vitamin needs.

Digestion begins in the mouth. The second rule for healthy eating is to chew your food until it is literally predigested in the mouth. Many abdominal disorders can be traced to gulping food. Eating quickly without paying attention to it is another cause of false appetite. Many people consume enormous amounts and still feel psychologically dissatisfied because they didn't fully realize the satisfaction of having eaten. The tendency then is to eat again in a short while.

A famous dietitian, when asked by an overweight patient for the best exercise to lose weight, answered, "Turn your head to the right, then turn your head to the left." He went on to explain to the bewildered woman, "When you are offered food from the right, turn your head to the left; when you are offered food from the left, turn your head to the right." Moderation in eating, when combined with selectivity in foods, proper preparation, and adequate mastication will create a balanced and wholesome diet and efficient digestion and elimination. Some consideration should also be given to fasting.

It is very important occasionally to give the digestive organs a chance to rest. Twenty-four hours of fasting produces a beneficial effect on almost anyone. A Russian doctor, N. Asimov, reported some startling evidence about prolonged fasting in a hospital experiment: In the patients treated by fasting, high blood pressure was normalized, as was coronary insufficiency—all within fifteen days. I, and many of my students, practice a twenty-four-hour fast once a week. Once a month, the fasting period is stretched either to thirty-six hours or even to two full days. Once a season, the purification fast described earlier is recommended.

Fasting is not only a physical discipline; it is always a great spiritual experience. We should prepare for fasting by some form of meditation that helps us to rid ourselves of any tendencies toward self-pity or unhappiness, partly because these emotions are not harmonious with the mental effects produced by fasting and partly because they may cause the fast to end in an orgy of eating to appease them. If properly prepared for, a day of fasting can be an exhilarating experience.

Fasting is a dramatic and highly effective way to begin a program of rejuvenation through diet. Through fasting for a brief time, eating habits can be completely reshaped, with the practicer returning to much healthier and more moderate habits. Of course, an older person, especially if he has any physical ailment, should consult a doctor before beginning a modified diet of any kind. Still, most of the guidelines given here will apply safely to anyone.

In the yoga tradition, diet is always a factor in treating ailments. More and more physicians are beginning to treat illnesses with diet prescriptions; some of the results are highly impressive. Recently, some discoveries of the relationship between diet and heart disease were reported by researchers at the Longevity Research Institute in Santa Barbara, California. According to them, people in advanced stages of angina, confined to wheelchairs, experienced dramatic recovery within a month of beginning therapy with a diet that is essentially cholesterol-free. One patient, a physician who was in agonizing pain when he entered the institute, began, within thirty days, to walk seventeen miles per day. One of the doctors who specializes in preventive medicine said, "If everybody with heart disease in the U.S. went on the diet tomorrow and stuck to it, 98 percent of the million-or-so Americans who will die of heart disease in the next year would be saved. And 80 percent would be free of heart disease at the end of a year."[1]

1. Reported in *New Woman*, Nov.–Dec. 1976, pp. 82–83.

8

Shaping the Body

> There is no beast, flower, or star as beautiful as the human
> body in its right form.
>
> —Eastern poet

In shaping the body there is a logical sequence of steps
that should begin with finding and maintaining one's correct weight. Extra poundage impedes progress in other
aspects of the program. Much of the program can be
carried out while shedding extra weight, but one should
begin there if necessary. I speak mainly of excessive
weight here rather than excessive thinness because the
former is a far more prevalent problem.[1] Of course, one
should also try to add weight if that is appropriate. And
if one is so fortunate as to have no weight problems,
one should take care to see that they don't develop.

The second focal point of this chapter is on posture,
another area of difficulty for many people who have gotten "out of shape." Then we move to body sculpting,
an art that is little known in the West except among a

---

1. A recent headline on one of those publications you find everywhere on
supermarket stands proclaimed that 70,000,000 Americans are overweight
(*The Star*, Feb. 2, 1978).

small group of body builders (where the concept of shaping the body is rather narrow and mechanical). There is also the important process of regaining suppleness wherever it has been lost in the process of aging. Finally, perhaps the greatest challenge lies in adjusting the inner life of the body—maintaining efficiency of blood circulation, digestion, and elimination, as well as metabolism.

Finding and Maintaining Appropriate Weight

One of the most frequent problems associated with aging is increased body weight and consequent loss of shape and vitality. Contrary to what many people believe and what most people experience as "inevitable," it is not necessary to "get out of shape" by increasing (or decreasing) one's weight as one grows older. In rare cases of sickness from disease or accident, a change in weight may be unavoidable. However, the aging process itself should not be blamed for changes in weight; the maintenance of a healthy body weight is one's own responsibility. The best time to assume that responsibility is before any change occurs, while one enjoys a good shape and weight.

There is an incredible joy in inhabiting the same body at age sixty as one inhabited at age twenty or twenty-five. The normally healthy person can stay in the same shape and possess the same weight throughout a lifetime. And, of course, many health problems that derive from excessive weight can be cured by weight loss. Conscientious men and women can enjoy the physical and mental well-being that comes by staying in shape as they grow older or, if necessary, getting back into shape after losing it. It is possible, even in cases of severe overweight, to regain one's youthful shape and size.

For people with acute weight problems, getting back

into shape is an experience that requires effort and some sacrifices, but in one sense it offers great rewards: The feeling of rejuvenation is powerful. Every weight problem has to be approached on an individual basis. In cases of obesity a physician should certainly be consulted before beginning a weight loss program. Hospitalization is sometimes recommended for severe cases. For most people, however, the principle of "do it yourself" will work satisfactorily, provided an intelligent approach is used. For chronically overweight people, the battle to lose weight is always long and arduous. But becoming a new person (and that is just what happens) is surely worth the discipline. Moreover, acquiring discipline can be a highly enjoyable experience once your mental and physical energies are dedicated to it.

One of the easiest ways to tell whether you are overweight (in a society of overweight people, the "average" is not a good guide) is to administer the pinch test I described earlier (see p. 11). Minor excesses can be dieted away rather easily. For those with more severe problems the pinch test is also a place to begin.

One way to focus on your weight is to take a scientific attitude toward the problem. You can begin by weighing every morning under the same conditions, after elimination and before eating breakfast. The scales will tell you day by day whether your present diet is appropriate or inappropriate. In cases of fluctuating weight, it is easy to adjust the caloric intake. Before and after festive seasons, holidays, or weekends when most of us tend to take in greater amounts of food or foods higher in calories than our weekday diet, one should be especially diligent to balance that extra amount of calories by taking fewer than one needs for a few days before or afterward, or occasionally by fasting.

A reducing program should always include muscle-toning exercises to prevent the body from losing its firmness, as well as exercises (*asanas* and *mudras*) for maintaining or increasing suppleness, more efficient blood circulation, and better digestion and elimination. While the body is slowly regaining its correct shape, its inner life must be gradually adjusted as well.

Begin your program of reshaping the body with an honest and well-informed assessment of your body weight: What does the pinch test tell you? What do your scales tell you? Are you willing to come to terms with your dietary habits? Are you ready for the adventure of discovering the new and youthful body that may presently be hidden from your outer eyes but which can be imagined and shaped into a reality? Then design a procedure for weight loss or gain that will bring that ideal body out of seclusion.

Improving Posture

The matter of improving posture can be carried on conjointly with a diet, whenever a diet is necessary. Otherwise, one can begin with it. Poor posture often consists of carrying the head awkwardly or perpetually raising the shoulders and hunching them in a stiff and unnatural manner. The stomach often leans forward, increasing the curve in the small of the back. Many people walk ungracefully and unnaturally. Some men especially tend to walk with their feet pointed outward in a kind of "Charlie Chaplin" gait, while others point their toes inward as they move.

Recently there has been a lot of discussion among psychologists about the relationship between posture and mental health. There is speculation that the stresses of modern life, among other things, cause many people to acquire tightness in various regions of the body, so that the posture becomes a reflection of an unconscious fear of being "punched in the stomach," for instance, or perhaps of an unconscious tendency to "bear the burdens of the world" on one's shoulders. We need not speculate here whether improved mental health leads to improved posture, but we can suggest that work on one's posture, if successful, will lead to a more positive mental attitude.

The procedure for adjusting posture should begin as before, with a detached look at oneself in front of a mirror. Then a series of exercises can help one to find and keep a natural, graceful way of sitting, standing, and moving.

To find the right position for the head, you can manipulate your neck in a circular movement until you see and sense the most appropriate relationship of head to shoulders. You may have to begin by adjusting the shoulders. One good method for doing so is to raise the shoulders as high as possible and then drop them into a relaxed position. Then bring the shoulders back as far as possible and return them to a relaxed position. Regular practice of these two movements of shoulders and head will improve their carriage in a short time.

Begin adjusting the middle part of the body by placing the right hand on the stomach and the left hand, palm out, on the area just below the small of the back (sacrum). Standing sideways to the mirror, manipulate the middle part of the body by gently drawing in the stomach while flattening the small of the back at the same time. Carry this posture in your sitting, standing, and walking.

Notice how you walk. Toes should point forward, and the feet and legs should carry the body's weight in balance. Another good exercise is to stand with your back against a wall, with heels, buttocks, shoulder blades, and back of the head touching the wall. Then walk away from the wall, retaining the sensation of being in correct balance.

The carriage of the entire body is improved by stretching. Standing straight, with the arms at the sides, stretch, trying to increase your height by a quarter of an inch. Then relax. The exercise should be repeated about half a dozen times. Apart from improving posture, this movement checks one important manifestation of aging, the tendency of the body to shrink with the passage of years.

Another exercise involves the combination of two opposite movements. Standing straight, one's height is first decreased by compressing the body to gain momentum for the next movement, which is a quick stretching upward as far as possible. Repeat half a dozen times.

In the East I learned of the belief that everyone is capable of increasing height, providing a sustained effort is made for a period of not less than ninety-nine days, with the stretching movements done at exactly the same time every day. The cycle of stretching exercises should terminate in "thinking tall," in which one stands very still, creating an image of oneself as a taller person.

Sculpting the Body

Improving the posture leads to the next discipline, which I call body sculpting. I learned about sculpting the body in old treatises of the Chinese Academy of Beauty, an ancient institution which was active during the Golden Age of Chinese culture (500–220 B.C.). In this institution, boys and girls were transformed into "walking flowers" by Chinese and Tibetan teachers who trained them and then sent them to the court of the ruling emperor to "please his heavenly eyesight." These young people received instruction in spiritual and physical disciplines. In addition, they learned how to write poetry, to sing, to dance, and to play musical instruments. Their physical training was not unlike rather elaborate isometric exercises, in which every group of muscles in the human body is tensed and relaxed a prescribed number of times. During this procedure they were taught to sculpt their bodies in their minds as they practiced breath control and exercise.

The human body has about 600 different groups of muscles, and if they are exercised regularly, firmness can be retained for a long time. Lack of exercise leads to flabbiness of the muscles, even atrophy, and, of course, deterioration of the shape. At any age one can considerably improve the contours of the body by using the muscle-toning techniques described below.

For our program here I have selected eighty-four slow movements for twelve major regions of the body. This cycle will take no more than five to seven minutes, but its regular practice makes an enormous difference in the appearance and strength of the body. It must be done with discipline every morning at the same time. Each movement is done seven times, slowly, with full concentration and with breath control. The best way to practice this cycle is in front of the mirror, either nude or in a bikini, so that the interplay of the muscles can be observed by the practicer. All these exercises are done in the standing position, starting with the arms and shoulders and moving downward to the calves and ankles. Focusing on one after another group of muscles, you shape your body in very much the same way as an artist sculpts a statue. Michelangelo liked to think that as he worked he was freeing a lovely form from a mass of stone. We can think of our work on the body in the same way. We are freeing our ideal form from whatever misproportions imprison it.

EXERCISE 1 (for biceps and shoulders)
    With feet slightly apart, arms stretched sideways at shoulder level with palms turned up, inhale while slowly bending arms toward the shoulders and tensing muscles

of the arms; exhale and return them to the original position and relax.

EXERCISE 2 (for forearms and chest)

With arms down at the sides, palms facing forward and keeping elbows pressed to the sides of the body, inhale while raising the forearms as if lifting a heavy barbell, making closed fists at the same time; with exhalation, lower forearms to the original position and open fists.

EXERCISE 3 (sides and back)

With arms stretched horizontally sideways, palms facing floor, inhale while exerting slow pressure downward, as if pushing against the air, tensing muscles at the sides of the body. Retain breath for a moment, then exhale while relaxing tension. Movement completed, it is repeated, again following the same pattern of breathing.

EXERCISE 4 (upper part of chest)

With arms extended forward parallel to each other, palms facing the floor, inhale while exerting powerful pressure downward, resulting in the tension of the chest muscles. Hold breath briefly, then relax while exhaling.

EXERCISE 5 (entire chest)

With inhalation, the arms are slowly raised from the sides to above the head while fists are closed. Then, with the right fist on top of the left, a downward pulling movement is practiced, as if pulling a taut rope, again tensing muscles of the chest and shoulders. This and the previous movement are especially recommended for women, as they exercise groups of muscles in the upper part of the chest which support the breasts. A youthful bustline can be retained by regular practice of this exercise.

EXERCISE 6 (chest, stomach, and back)

Standing with feet slightly apart, hands clasped (palms together) in front at chest level, while inhaling push the right hand against the left, resisting with the left but moving both hands to the left, tensing chest muscles. Relax with exhalation. Repeat the same movement to the right side.

EXERCISE 7 (chest, shoulders, and back)

Standing with the fists pressed together at the chest level, elbows pointing out, with inhalation slowly move the fists apart as if pulling a heavy spring. Relax with exhalation. Strong pressure is exerted between the shoulder blades.

EXERCISE 8 (chest expansion, back, and buttocks)

With the feet wide apart, arms extended forward, fists closed, inhale while pulling the arms sideways and apart. The whole body bends slightly backward until tension in the muscles of the back and the buttocks is felt. With exhalation, arms are returned to the original position.

EXERCISE 9 (abdomen)

Fingertips are placed on the region of the abdomen. With inhalation, the abdominal muscles are tensed; with exhalation, they are relaxed. Here, the muscles are tensed in very much the same way as when having a bowel movement.

EXERCISE 10 (thighs)

Concentration is on the thighs. Knees are slightly bent and then thigh muscles are tensed as you straighten the legs on inhalation. Relax with exhalation.

EXERCISE 11 (calves)

With inhalation the body is raised on the tip of the toes while tensing the muscles of the calves. Exhale while relaxing.[2]

EXERCISE 12 (all muscle groups)

The last exercise in this cycle is know as the "key" exercise. This exercise is done in a standing position. Every muscle of the body is slowly tensed with inhalation, including closing of hands into fists, and relaxed with exhalation. During the tensing an idealized self-image— youthful and healthy—is projected onto the screen of one's imagination. This is the most important among the exercises.[3]

Practicing every exercise slowly for seven times and at the same time of the morning is extremely important for people past their fifties. In fact, the older a person gets, the more importance should be placed on this cycle of exercises because, as people get older, muscles tend to be exercised less and less. Even after two weeks of regular practice, the change in muscle tone is visible, and one experiences the sensation of increased strength. The seven repetitions are minimal to achieve beneficial results, but in the case of long neglect of the muscles, fourteen or even twenty-one repetitions should be practiced on a regular basis.

2. According to a tradition I learned in China, movement on the tip of your toes is one of the nine basic movements of the human body. The others are six movements of the spine (forward, backward, to the right, to the left, twisting to the right and left), a stretching movement with the arms up, as if trying to reach an object high above the head, and squatting. Moving on tiptoes not only develops the muscles of the calves but keeps feet (instep and ankles) in a healthy condition.

3. Modern research suggests that this exercise, modified in the following manner, could normalize blood pressure in a fairly short time: Every muscle of the body is tensed, but fists are not closed; instead of retaining breath, it flows naturally in and out during tension.

Besides these muscular movements for twelve groups of muscles in the main regions of the body, there is a cycle especially for the abdominal muscles. The middle of the human body is the most treacherous in losing shape. That is where the deterioration starts with 99 people out of 100. In aging a once beautiful, flat, and well-molded abdomen becomes paunchy; the waistline increases from two inches up to twelve or more. The change is meekly accepted by most people as "an unavoidable manifestation of aging." Yet the change is perfectly avoidable with a bit of willpower and self-discipline.

Here is a threefold test for your abdomen. Lying flat on your back, with the hands alongside the body, try to sit up, keeping your heels on the floor. If you succeed, try sitting up with the arms folded on the chest, and if this effort is positive, try to do the same with the hands clasped behind the neck. This simple test will give you a fairly accurate assessment of the condition of your abdominal muscles.

Five to ten minutes should be spent daily toning up and strengthening these abdominal muscles to avoid sinking into shapelessness. Most of the exercises are done in the supine position. In the yogic tradition, these exercises are done with breath control, inhaling as you exert effort and exhaling as you relax.

EXERCISE 1

Lying in the supine position, with inhalation the legs are lifted up to a 45-degree angle; with exhalation, they are lowered to the original position. Repeat 6 times.

EXERCISE 2

Lying as before, with inhalation draw the knees up to the stomach and stretch them upward at right angles to the body; with exhalation slowly lower them, controlling the movement with the muscles of the stomach. Repeat 6 times.

EXERCISE 3 (not for people with high blood pressure)

In a supine position, knees are slowly raised to the stomach with inhalation, clasped by the hands, and pressed tightly to the stomach with retention of breath for 3–4 heartbeats. Then legs are lowered as breath is exhaled. Repeat 4 times.

This exercise is not only good for abdominal muscles; it removes gases from the stomach and produces a powerful flushing effect on the brain. In yoga it is considered one of the techniques to improve memory.

EXERCISE 4

Lying as before, the legs are separated as they are raised to the sides with inhalation, describing a circle. At the high point they are brought together and then lowered onto the floor with exhalation. Repeat 4–6 times.

EXERCISE 5

Lying as before, with inhalation, knees are slowly brought to the stomach, then legs are stretched upward, raising the upper part of the body at the same time so that you are balanced on your buttocks. For a moment the body assumes a V position while breath is retained; then body is slowly lowered to the original position while breath is exhaled. Repeat 4 times.

EXERCISE 6

Lie on your back, then prop up your upper torso with your elbows; on inhalation, with legs stretched out in front, slowly raise and lower legs in a scissors movement, not touching the floor with the feet, and letting the stomach feel the stress. Exhale while relaxing. Repeat 3–4 times.

EXERCISE 7

Sitting up in a cross-legged position, arms folded on the chest, inhale while straightening arms and legs as the body inclines slightly backward. Repeat until a slight tiredness is felt.

The sit-ups described as preliminary trials are wonderful movements to tone up and strengthen the abdominal muscles. Depending upon the physical condition of the practicer, they can be done in any of the three positions described for the arms.

Above all, a means of toning up abdominal muscles is to practice *uddiyan,* flapping *uddiyan,* and *nauli* (see pp. 85–87), exercises that are the epitome of abdominal control.

In cases of gross obesity of the stomach, the exercises alone will not rectify the problem. A wise diet should be considered as well. However, the exercises are very important to prevent and correct flabbiness in abdominal muscles.

Regaining Suppleness

With the passage of years the body tends to become progressively rigid. Checking this process and then reversing it is a great victory over time. Many students who experience this victory testify to a sensation of youth. With the regaining of suppleness, the biological clock is turned backward. Suppleness is alien to old age in the experience of most people. Reversing the progressive stiffness of the body is a long and strenuous battle requiring a lot of dedication and willpower.

A great number of yoga *asanas* are designed to achieve suppleness. Prior to executing them you should spend five to ten minutes warming up the body in very much the same way a runner or jumper warms up prior to engaging in sports events. One should not be too ambitious, avoiding at all costs possible injury, straining the muscles, or overtaxing the joints. In the beginning one must be satisfied with a little progress.

In the following program to regain suppleness, I have selected a number of movements from Taoist yoga and have designed some movements myself to harmonize with modern Western exercises. The first group are warm-up exercises for shoulder blades, spine, and joints of the upper body.

EXERCISE 1

In a standing position, the shoulders should be rotated together in a circular movement, first backward, then forward, 4 times in each direction.

EXERCISE 2

One of the most important exercises is to rotate each shoulder separately in a movement not unlike that of the backstroke swimmer. One shoulder moves forward while the other moves backward. The body follows the movement of the shoulders, swaying slightly back and forth and from side to side. Although the movements are done with the shoulders, the exercise is predominantly for the spine, as each vertebra is pivoted, one upon the other, in its socket.

The faculty of the mind's eye or the ability to "look into oneself" plays a most important part in this exercise. Traditionally, the movement is done with eyes closed, gradually increasing awareness of one's inner body. These two exercises above not only contribute to the suppleness of the shoulder blades but increase the flow of arterial blood to the roots of the spinal nerves, stimulating the sympathetic nervous system.

The following exercises will limber up the small of the back.

EXERCISE 3

Both arms should be stretched up and worked in a hand-over-hand movement as if one were climbing a ladder. When you can't stretch further, let yourself fall forward from the waist, with the aim of touching the floor with the tips of your fingers. The upper part of the body should be completely relaxed, but with legs straight and stiff. The movement, if done correctly, should produce a stretching sensation at the back of the legs as well as in the ligaments attached to the spinal cord.

People with high blood pressure should avoid the movements below that require bending down, as this increases the flow of blood to the head. For others, this movement has the additional benefit of helping to delay wrinkles through increased blood circulation in the skin and tissues of the face.

EXERCISE 4

Standing with the feet apart as before, hands down, let the upper part of the body, in a relaxed but strong rhythmical movement, lean forward 3 times, trying to touch the floor with the tips of the fingers. After you have performed this movement several times, stretch the raised body to the left, then to the right, and eventually backward. The cycle is completed by relaxed rotary movement of the trunk 4 times left to right and 4 times right to left, until a sensation of warmth and suppleness

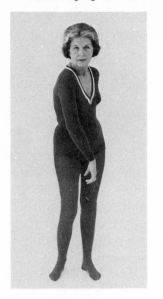
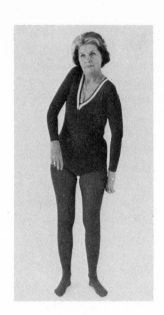

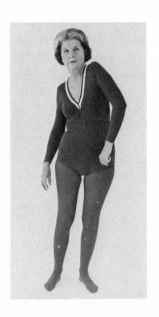
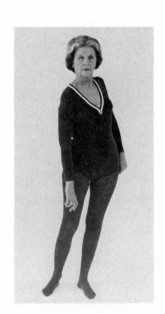

is achieved. This is an excellent warming-up exercise cycle prior to executing the *asanas.*

To assess one's condition in regard to suppleness, a simple three-part test can be taken: Seated on a comfortable mat or rug, both legs stretched forward, the right leg is brought close to the body, right hand securing a good grip on the right toe. While maintaining the grip, leg is slowly stretched forward until it is completely flat on the floor. The same is done with the left leg. In the next movement, the right leg again is brought close to the body, grip on toe secured, but instead of stretching it flat on the floor, it is stretched upward at a 45-degree angle. Repeat on the left side. As in the first movement, a complete stretch should be made. In the third test, the right foot is brought close to the body and then lifted with both arms while you sit straight, in an attempt to touch the forehead with the big toe. Again, repeat with the left leg.

If these three movements can be done without great difficulty, one's body is in a healthy state of suppleness. Most people, however, especially after age forty, will find great difficulty in passing this test. During the practice of regaining suppleness, these movements could always serve as a certain reference to one's progress.

The spinal column allows six basic movements: forward and backward, to the right and left, and twisting in opposite directions. There are bodily postures in yoga for each of these movements.

Forward-Stretching *Asanas*

EXERCISE 1

While sitting on a comfortable mat or rug, the right leg is bent toward the body and the foot placed under the left thigh. Knees are kept close to each other. Inhale with the back straight and bend forward, securing hold of a foot or an ankle; while exhaling, try to touch knee with forehead. Repeat once and then change position of the legs.

EXERCISE 2

Instead of placing foot underneath thigh, press it to the inside of the thigh and bend forward in the same manner.

EXERCISE 3

Instead of pressing foot to inside of thigh, it is placed flat on the floor close to the body, knee raised to a 45-degree angle that still permits you to bend forward.

EXERCISE 4

Sitting as before, left leg is extended forward while right foot is placed on top of the left thigh with the heel close to the groin, knee on floor. Movement and breathing are the same as before.

EXERCISE 5

This exercise consists of sitting cross-legged with back and neck straight and inhaling. Both hands are brought from the outside under thighs to grasp feet. Exhale as you bend forward between knees, with the objective of touching the floor with your forehead.

Backward-Bending *Asanas*

Backward-bending movements are very important for maintaining healthy condition of the spine. A number of preliminary movements can be practiced prior to executing *asanas;* seven of them are listed in chapter 14 on rebirth. In all these exercises, inhalation is done while effort is being made and exhalation while relaxing.

EXERCISE 1

In a standing position, feet apart, place hands on the hips, bend forward, and rock gently 3–4 times.

EXERCISE 2

Standing as above, with the back to the wall, raise hands over the head and place on the wall. In the beginning retain the position just for a few seconds, and later on attempt to walk down the wall with your hands.

EXERCISE 3

Lying on the stomach, place hands on the waist. The top part of the body is slowly raised with inhalation as high as possible, head brought back toward waist. Exhale and relax.

EXERCISE 4

Lying as before (on the stomach), raise legs together with the head and shoulders as you inhale. Pay special attention to the position of the legs, which are kept as straight as possible.

EXERCISE 5

Another excellent exercise for achieving suppleness is the pose of a cat. Standing on knees and hands and keeping elbows straight, bring stomach down with inhalation and raise head simultaneously so that you are looking forward. With exhalation, the position is reversed and the back is humped in the gesture of a cat stretching its spine. The position is beneficial for the healthy condition of the spine. One important aspect should be mentioned: With the movement of the abdomen down, the rectum is opened and slightly pushed out; with the movement up, it is drawn in and contracted. Since the rectum is the terminal point of the spinal nerve, the exercise serves as a powerful toning medium for the entire sympathetic nervous system, as well as a stimulating movement for the sphincters of the rectum.

A variation of this exercise is especially beneficial in cases of persistent pain in the small of the back. While the stomach is protruded with inhalation, hips are swung to the right and then to the left while breath is retained; then breath is exhaled while back is humped or raised.

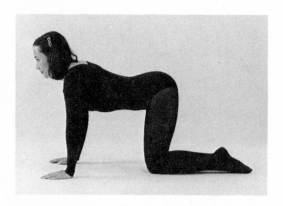

Pose of a cat—Inhalation

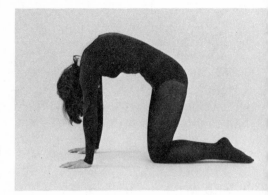

Pose of a cat—Exhalation

EXERCISE 6

The supine pelvic pose is performed while sitting between heels, body slowly lowered backward until back is completely flat. Hands are placed under the neck, rhythmical breath maintained.

EXERCISE 7

A pose closely related to the previous one is to sit on heels and practice the same movement backward until the crown of the head rests on the floor. Place hands in the attitude of prayer on the chest. Maintain rhythmical breath. In this position the small of the back is greatly arched.

Twisting of the Spine

As with the backward-bending positions, preliminary exercises involving twisting of the spine should be practiced before going on to the more demanding *asanas* given in chapter 14 on rebirth.

EXERCISE 1

In a standing position with feet apart, stretch arms sideways. Maintain the position of the hips, and slowly twist the body to the right and to the left with mind concentrated on rotary movements in every socket of the spinal column.

EXERCISE 2

Standing as above, stretch arms to the sides and then bend at elbows. Movements are done vigorously, rather than slowly, from side to side.

EXERCISE 3

Standing as above, bend body forward until it is parallel with the floor, arms extended sideways. With exhalation, twist body to the left, right arm trying to touch left toe, and raise to repeat on the other side.

EXERCISE 4

Spinal twist (preliminary): Seated with the legs stretched forward, place right foot on the other side of the left knee. With exhalation, twist body to the left in one strong movement until each vertebra is rotated in its socket. Movement is repeated on the other side (with legs changing positions also).

EXERCISE 5: Pose of a Serpent

Lying on the stomach, place hands near the shoulders, palms down. With inhalation, the top part of the body is slowly raised, leaving the lower part of the stomach around the navel in contact with the floor. In the process of raising the body, head and shoulders are twisted to the right with the aim of attaining a clear look at the left heel. Exhale as you return to the original position, then repeat movement while twisting to the left for a look at the right heel. In this movement, vertebrae of the spine are twisted to the left and to the right and the spine is arched backward.

EXERCISE 6: Half of the Locust

Lying flat on the stomach, hands alongside the body, raise the right leg as high as possible with inhalation and lower with exhalation. Same repeated with the left leg.

Movements to the Right and Left

Sideways movements of the spine must be practiced regularly to completely regain suppleness in the backbone. Preliminary movements for this purpose include forcing the body sideways in a rhythmical swing of one arm at a time over the head to assist the sideways swing of the upper torso. Body should be bent 2–3 times before returning to standing position with feet apart. Do this as many times as needed to "limber up."

EXERCISE 1

Standing with the feet apart and arms stretched outward to the sides at shoulder level, inhale. Right leg is bent at knee while body moves to right, with outstretched arms turning vertically to place right palm on the floor. Exhalation is combined with sideways movement. Movement is repeated on the other side.

EXERCISE 2

Sideways swing. Sitting on the floor on a comfortable mat or rug, raise arms and lock hands at wrists while bending both legs at the knees to the right side of the body. Inhalation is done while torso is straight; with exhalation, body is rocked toward the feet several times. Perform 2–3 times on one side before changing position of legs and direction of the stretch.

EXERCISE 3

Sit with one leg stretched forward, only one leg bent sideways. Hands with fingers interlaced rest on the head. After deep inhalation, move body sideways with the aim of bringing the elbow as close as possible to the floor. With legs changed, repeat movement on the other side.

A more demanding *asana* known as Pose of a Dove is included in chapter 14 on rebirth.

9

Care of the Face and Head

Signs of age often appear first in the area of the head: graying, thinning, and brittle hair; lines, wrinkles, and sags in the face and chin; failing eyesight; deterioration of teeth and gums. This chapter is designed to help you retard these marks of aging through hygiene, exercise, and special treatment. We will focus on one area at a time.

Facial Exercises

If the muscles of the body are not exercised on a regular basis, they deteriorate and the body loses its shape. The same thing can be said about the muscles of the face. Very often, detrimental changes in the contour of the face occur because the facial muscles are not exercised at all, even by hard chewing. Leading cosmeticians now recognize that regular practice of facial exercises, especially after the age of forty, can delay deterioration of the facial tissues.

The passage of time affects first the muscles and then the tissues of the face. There are a number of reasons for that. The face is exposed to the elements; blood circulation is often not adequate in skin and tissues of the face; stress and worry leave their marks on it. One of the greatest enemies of facial beauty is gravitational pull, which causes the contour of the face to change and the corners of the mouth to sag, as well as the muscles of cheeks and chin. Muscles of the face are rarely exercised. Our diet, especially for elderly people, is getting softer and mushier, eliminating the natural exercise that could be achieved through good chewing.

People's faces do not age in a uniform way. Some people are affected in the neck, others in the lips and mouth, others in the cheek muscles, others in the forehead, around the eyes, along the nose to mouth, giving them a sad expression, like a Greek tragic mask. It is really remarkable how signs of aging can be improved or prevented in most cases without plastic surgery. It requires great perseverance, dedication, and knowledge as well as an unfailing belief in ultimate success.

On numerous occasions I have observed a more youthful appearance emerge through the discipline of bodily and facial exercises. A number of my students have reported the gradual disappearance of brown age spots concurrent with a general improvement in their looks, all as a result of exercise. This phenomenon is also described by some plastic surgeons who report that after a successful face-lift they saw the disappearance of age spots in parts of the body unrelated to surgery. My explanation is that the mind is delighted and pleased by the change in one's appearance so that it reprograms the body in some yet unknown manner to change its chemistry.

The history of the first facial exercises can be traced to the ancient treatises of the Chinese Academy of Beauty. In the island ashram of my Chinese master who was engaged in work with elderly people, special exercises were practiced twice daily, in many cases with astonishing results. Thinking about this experience, I realize now that in some cases the prolonged effect of facial exercises was the equivalent of, or perhaps even better than, plastic surgery.

In the ashram there was a tradition of shaving the hair on the head on a regular basis. There were, of course, no electric shavers or even safety razors, and this painful procedure was carried out by hand, wielding a razor-sharp switchblade (using little or no soap) as it was done 2,000 years ago. I never enjoyed the operation; nevertheless, by observing the interplay of muscles on the shining skulls of my brothers in yoga I learned many facial exercises, a number of which were designed to counteract gravitational pull.

Below I describe fifteen exercises related to fifteen groups of muscles. Besides these, inverted positions, such as the half shoulder stand, the pose of longevity, the half head pose, the yin/yang pose, and the full headstand should be practiced on a regular basis to counteract gravitational pull and direct a flow of arterial blood to the skin and tissues of the face.

Prior to embarking on facial exercises, the face should be studied in front of a mirror in a detached and critical manner. An overall plan should be made to achieve the best results from exercise. Some people should concentrate on the region commonly known as the "double chin," whereas others should emphasize exercises for the mouth; still others should pay more attention to eyes and forehead. Facial exercises are done from the neck up, gradually working on the mouth, cheeks, eyes, forehead, and scalp.

EXERCISE 1
Sitting in a cross-legged position, raise the head as high as possible, then open the mouth and slowly close it, with the lower lip overlapping the top lip. The final

position is retained for a few seconds, then the chin is relaxed and the exercise is repeated. 4 times.

EXERCISE 2
Open the mouth partially and tense the muscles of the neck and throat for a few seconds, then relax. 4 times.

EXERCISE 3
Inhale through the mouth, forming the letter *o:* Cheeks are drawn in, creating dimples on either side. Breath is exhaled through the mouth while cheeks are slightly puffed and lips relaxed. 6 times or more.

EXERCISE 4
With fists on top of each other, place them under the chin, exerting pressure. Open and close mouth against this pressure in the manner of a breathing fish (lips pursed). 4 times.

EXERCISE 5
A small amount of air is inhaled into the mouth. Using it as a ball, push it under the top lip, bottom lip, right and left cheeks vigorously for a minute or so.

EXERCISE 6
This exercise is a little more difficult; nevertheless, it can be learned in a very short time. In the beginning it can be practiced in front of a mirror.

The left thumb is placed into the mouth while four fingers of the left hand press against the cheek on the outside. In that position, try to smile with the right part of your mouth against the pressure of the thumb and four fingers. You are resisting with the pressure of your thumb and fingers your attempt to smile. The muscles are exercised against pressure. After resting for a few seconds, use the right hand to exercise the left side of the face in the same manner. Exercise can be repeated 3–4 times on each side.

EXERCISE 7

Inhale through the nose. Place three fingers of the left hand at the left corner of the mouth and three fingers of the right hand at the right corner of the mouth. Exhale in short bursts through pursed lips, at the same time exerting pressure with the fingers against the corners of the mouth. 4 times.

EXERCISE 8

Placing index and middle finger at the sides of the face, exert gentle but firm pressure as you tense and relax your cheeks alternatively. Try not to puff your cheeks, but feel with your fingers that you are exercising the muscles of the cheeks (not stretching the skin). 4 times.

EXERCISE 9

Place the index and middle finger on your eyebrows, pressing them to the skull. When pressure is exerted, try to raise your eyebrows. Relax and repeat 4 times. In this exercise, muscles of the forehead as well as muscles of the top eyelid are toned up.

EXERCISE 10

Press index fingers tightly at the outer corner of the eyes. Eyes are closed, pressure exerted, then the eyes closed more tightly, relaxed, again closed tightly, relaxed and so on, 4–6 times. This exercise stimulates and tones the skin where crow's feet appear at the corners of the eyes.

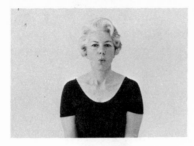

For lips—
Inhalation

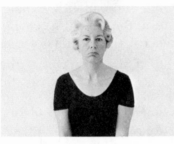

For lips—
Exhalation

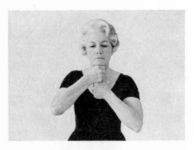

For double chin

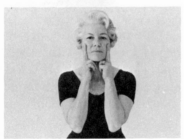

For lips and cheeks

EXERCISE 11

This exercise is very simple and could be practiced in front of a mirror. Open the eyes slowly as wide as posible; retain position for 2 seconds, and then slowly close eyes tighter and tighter. To finish the exercise, open eyes and blink quickly a few times. 4 times.

EXERCISE 12

Three fingers of each hand are placed on closed eyelids in such a manner: Index finger presses on the outside corner of the eye; middle finger presses the middle of the eyebrow; ring finger creates gentle pressure on the inner corners of the eyes. In that position, with gentle pressure created by all three fingers, close eyes tightly; relax pressure. 4 times.

EXERCISE 13

This and the following exercises are demanding because they include the semivoluntary muscles of the skull. The easiest way to learn how to do them is in front of a mirror. For the first one, keeping the face perfectly calm, without moving any other group of muscles, contract the muscles of the skull, trying to achieve an effect in which the entire face is lifted ⅛ of an inch or so against gravitational pull. If done correctly, the result is a smoothing of the horizontal wrinkles of the forehead and the movement of both ears upward. It is felt to be essentially like face-lift surgery. The movement should be felt even under the chin. When the entire face is lifted properly, the final position should be retained for one or two seconds, then the face is slowly relaxed. 4 times.

EXERCISE 14

This exercise is even more demanding. It consists of tensing the muscles at the back of the skull, resulting

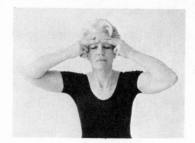

For lines between
the eyebrows

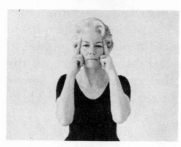

For crow's feet

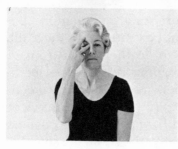

For eyelids

Pose of a Lion
(*Simhasana*)

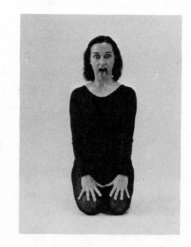

in a gentle stretch of the face horizontally. When mastered, both ears move closer to the skull and vertical lines in the face are smoothed out.

EXERCISE 15 Pose of a Lion *(Simhasana)*

A good all-around facial exercise, known also as one of the techniques of longevity, is the famous pose of a lion of Indian yoga. In this exercise not only every muscle of the face is toned up and stimulated, but the root of the tongue, the mouth, and the throat are exercised as well. Traditionally, it is done while sitting on the back of the heels, back and neck in a straight line, arms stretched, hands resting on the knees. After deep inhalation through the nose, the arms, shoulders, and chest muscles are tensed as much as possible, fingers are spread apart, and eyes opened as wide as possible. Mouth is wide open, too, and tongue is pushed out of the mouth as far as possible. The position creates a powerful tension in the top part of the body. It should be retained for 3–4 seconds. Then every muscle is relaxed as the face is returned to its relaxed position. After a few seconds, the position is repeated. This exercise is considered so powerful that only 4 repetitions are done at one sitting.

In Chinese museums I saw ancient vases depicting young maidens patting their faces and dancing with their arms lifted up, singing, "Men are coming, cheeks are rosy, hands are white." Patting of the face with the fingertips is perhaps the oldest beauty exercise in the world.

In yoga, the fingertips are used extensively in stimulating and relaxing facial muscles. After a set of facial exercises is finished, the face is gently tapped with the fingertips, starting from the forehead and moving downward to cheeks and around the mouth. These up and down movements are repeated several times until the sensation of pleasant warmth is achieved in the skin of the face.

The final practice is complete relaxation of the facial muscles, known in yogic tradition as "releasing of the inner light." The phenomenon of the face becoming enlightened has been known in Western traditions as well as in Eastern ones: "She walked into the room with her face lit up." Or "The moment he reached the decision his face lit up." And so on. I believe that at the moment of complete relaxation, the inner beauty of a person, often hidden and obscured by the mask of tension, starts to shine through. Tension can be erased by the gentle movement of the fingertips to smooth areas of tension.

On Saturdays the ashram of one of my Chinese teachers was open to people with a variety of problems. My teacher was also a well-known healer. I remember how on one Saturday morning an elderly woman walked into the community room of the ashram and sat down in a corner in the meek attitude of a person defeated by life. She sat quietly with her head inclined to one side. The story of her unhappy life was written on her aged face. The teacher entered and spotted her at once. He walked straight to her, knelt in front of her, and started to talk to her in a kind and reassuring voice. "Don't worry, don't worry," he said to her. "Life is not ended. Everything will change for the better soon." At the same time he started to stroke her face with light gestures of his long, exquisite fingers. I was watching them closely. A miracle happened in front of my eyes. He took twenty years off her face, as if with his fingers he had peeled off the mask of tension.

The exercise involving fingertips is done in front of a mirror. The face is studied and relaxed as much as possible. If there is any awareness that complete relaxation hasn't been achieved, a gentle touch of the fingers is applied to the region of the face where tension is still present, as if to help groups of muscles chronically tensed to relax completely.

Beauty Masks

In the treatises of the ancient academy of beauty mentioned previously, there are references to beauty masks. Amazingly enough, these beauty masks can be used today because they consist of natural ingredients. In fact, some are used in modern beauty salons, while others are still unknown to the general public. I would like to describe some of the least-known treatments.

Honey Masks

Honey was widely used in ancient times in a remarkable range of treatments. It was used to prevent and cure arthritis and rheumatism, kidney, liver, and stomach disorders, as a purifier of the entire system, and as a tonic during recuperation from various diseases. In combination with hot milk or tea it was used for sore throats, bronchitis, and various infections of the lungs. It was also widely used for external treatment to speed up healing of wounds and as a beauty mask. There are references to at least 100 varieties of honey in old Chinese pharmacological books. Below is a list of beauty masks containing honey.

In all these masks a natural, light-colored honey should be used. It is rich in vitamins C, B_2, B_6, and pantothenic acid. Do not apply the masks over extremely sensitive skin rashes or eczema. All these masks can be applied once or twice a week or even daily for a short period of time. The main purpose of these masks is rejuvenation of the skin through nourishment. In each case, cold water with lemon juice should be used to rinse the face.

1. *Honey and Milk*

One tablespoon of warm honey stirred with an equal amount of warm milk. After applying evenly to the skin of the face (previously cleaned with warm water or cleansing lotion), the mask is left on for 10 minutes and then removed with cold water and lemon juice. This mask is especially beneficial for dry and tired skin that shows signs of aging.

2. *Honey and Tea*

To treat oily skin, a tablespoon of honey can be mixed with an equal amount of warm, freshly prepared tea and applied as above.

3. *Honey, Egg Yolk, and Oil*

One egg yolk is stirred with a tablespoon of warm honey and a teaspoon of vegetable oil (corn, apricot, olive, or sunflower). After applying this mask evenly over face and neck, leave it on for 10 to 15 minutes, then wash off with cold water and lemon juice. This mask has a nourishing, stimulating, and rejuvenating effect on tired skin.

4. *Honey and Egg White*

One egg white is stirred with one teaspoon of warm honey. Application, duration, and removal are the same as above.

Egg Masks

The egg, a symbol of new life, was the next most popular rejuvenating and stimulating treatment for aging skin.

1. *Egg Mask*

A fresh egg is well mixed and applied evenly on the skin for 10–15 minutes. In cases of dry skin, prior to the application of this mask, soften the skin with pure vegetable oil. This mask is also a nourishing one. It tightens large pores and makes the skin tighter and younger looking.

2. *Egg White Mask*

Egg white is applied evenly over the face after the drier areas are softened with almond oil. Leave the mask on for 10 minutes and then remove with cotton wool and cold water. While drying, the egg white has a powerful toning effect on tired skin, makes small wrinkles less visible, and tightens enlarged pores. The powerful toning effect of the egg white was known in ancient China and became a base for many other masks.

3. *Egg White–Lemon Mask*

In this mask the white of one egg is beaten to the consistency of foam; during the beating a teaspoon of lemon juice is added drop by drop. The mask is left for the same duration as above and removed the same way. The addition of lemon juice gives this mask additional quality. It whitens the skin and bleaches and destroys blackheads. The general effect of this mask is refreshing and stimulating.

4. *Egg White–Berry Mask*

In this mask, instead of lemon juice use cranberry, raspberry, or strawberry juice in the same manner as previously. It was believed that the juice of red berries gives the skin a pleasant rosy tint, highly sought among Eastern women. Leave 10–15 minutes.

Milk-Based Masks

Rinsing and washing the face in milk, especially goat's milk, is one of the oldest beauty treatments known from Peking to Rome, Kiev to London. After the face is carefully washed with water which is softened with baking soda, it is washed again in milk, which is left to dry on the face. After 10–15 minutes, the face is cleaned with a cleansing lotion.

Cottage Cheese Mask

For normal and dry skin, 2 tablespoons of cottage cheese are stirred with a tablespoon of sour cream or milk. For oily skin, instead of milk or sour cream, an equal amount of yogurt is used. The mask is left on the skin for 15 minutes, washed off with warm water, and then rinsed with cold water. Because of the presence of sour milk acid and vitamins, this mask softens, cleans, and whitens the skin. It also tones and tightens aging skin. It is especially recommended in cases of brown age spots. It can also be used for hands with the same problem.

Fruit, Berry, and Vegetable Masks

These masks are most recommended for skin which has lost its youthful firmness.

1. Turnip or Horseradish Mask

Grated turnip or horseradish is blended to a creamy consistency. It must be mixed more or less equally with sour cream, and special care should be exercised to avoid contact with the eyes. It can be applied either directly to the face and neck or laid first on a clean piece of linen with holes for eyes, nose, and mouth. Mask should remain on skin for only 5–10 minutes. Then carefully wash it off with cold water, lemon juice added. This mask has a great toning effect on the skin and can be used every second day for a period of two weeks; from then on, once or twice a week. These masks have been known to remove age spots and convey to the skin its original velvetlike quality.

2. *Avocado Mask*

Half a ripe avocado (mashed) is applied evenly over the face and left on for 10–15 minutes. Wash off with cold water. This mask has found its way into Western beauty culture and is widely used.

3. *Cranberry Mask*

This is especially popular in Chinese and Russian traditions. Ripe cranberries are blended into a creamy consistency and applied to the face. The mask is retained for 10–15 minutes and then washed off with cold water. Apart from a toning and vitalizing effect, regular application of this mask will greatly contribute to a rosy complexion. Strawberries are also used in this way (recommended for more delicate skin).

4. *Watermelon Treatment*

Outstanding among the above-mentioned beauty masks is the famous watermelon beauty treatment of China. After carefully cleansing the face, rub it with a piece of red melon. This treatment should always be done in sunny weather so that immediately after the application of watermelon, the face can be exposed to sunshine. Eyes closed, the face is slowly turned from side to side so that every part of it is uniformly exposed to sunlight. The treatment has a remarkable toning effect on the skin, improving complexion and firmness as well as removing age spots.

Neck and Eyes

I decided to put neck and eye exercises in the same section because, traditionally, neck exercises are done before eye exercises. It is believed that certain relaxed movements of the neck have a direct correlation with the eyesight and can lead to actual improvement of the eyesight as well as preventing deterioration of the eyes during the middle part of life.

Neck

Neck exercises are done in a cross-legged position in cycles of four movements. Breathing during the neck exercises is natural (i.e., no special breath control practiced).

1. Turn head to the right and then to the left, in a strong but not strained movement. 4 times.
2. Looking straight forward, tilt head toward the left shoulder and then to the right shoulder. 4 times.
3. Move head up and down as far in each direction as you can. 4 times.
4. Sitting straight, thrust the chin forward and then draw slowly back. Concentrate on the region of the double chin. 4 times.

5. Bring head up as high as possible, eyes closed, and then drop head to the chest in a completely relaxed movement. 4 times.

6. Sitting straight, rotate the head for half a circle toward the right and then drop to relax against the chest as in the previous exercise. Then rotate for half a circle in the other direction and drop forward from the back. 4 times.

   The emphasis in movements 5 and 6 is on complete relaxation. In the tradition of Taoist yoga, these two movements have a direct effect on the eyesight. They are always mentioned as exercises to help retain good sight in the late years of life.

7. Follow a slow and relaxed rotary movement 4 times clockwise and then 4 times counterclockwise.

Note: After finishing the neck exercises, massage the neck in two ways: First, bow the head and massage the nape of the neck by quick and gentle pats with the hands. In the second one, raise the head and pat the region under the chin with the back sides of the fingers.

Eyes

Upon completion of the neck exercises, you are ready for eye exercises. They are also done in a cross-legged seated position. They include various movements of the eyeballs to strengthen the ocular muscles and to train the eyes to see at different angles. The set of eye exercises involves not only movements of the eyeball but the ability to fix the gaze at predetermined points during the movements. After each movement, close and relax eyes for 10–15 seconds.

1. Looking up and then down. Each time you actually concentrate your gaze for a second on a chosen point: up, then down. 4 times.
2. After looking up, fix eyes straight forward, then down, and then again straight forward. 4 times.
3. Looking straight forward, bring eyes to the right and then to the left, right, left—fixing gaze each time at an object on the right and then the left. 4 times.
4. Same as 3, but pause in the middle each time.
5. Looking diagonally, right corner up, left corner down. Do not stop in center. 4 times. Then change to left corner up, right corner down. 4 times.
6. Focus eyes on the tip of the nose and then look straight forward. Close eyes. 4 times.
7. Changing focus. Index finger is brought in front of the face at the level of the eyes, usually to a distance that enables you to see the lines on your fingertip. Focus eyes for a few seconds on the fingertip. Then bring gaze forward and into the distance without focusing on any particular object. Focus and unfocus. The purpose is to alternate.
8. Here is an unusual eye exercise highly favored in Chinese yoga. Two index fingers are brought together on the level with the eyes and at a distance of 12 inches from the face. For a few seconds, concentrate focus between the fingers, then slowly raise it, looking over the fingers into the distance. At this point fingers are in a semifocus and a "third finger" appears between the fingertips. Eyes are brought back into the focus at the point between the fingers, destroying the illusion. Exercise is repeated 4 times.

9. Staring. The exercise is known as a restorer of the eyesight. It consists of an unblinking gaze directed to an object several feet in front of you. The purpose of this exercise is actually to see the object better at the end of half a minute's gaze. Eyes are then closed, relaxed, and exercise is repeated.

10. Rolling of the eyeballs slowly clockwise and counterclockwise without missing a single point in the space covered by your gaze. Your eyes should cover a circle made of thousands of points that you are scanning as you move the eyes along the circle. As in previous exercises, this one involves not only movement but an attempt to direct the gaze so that it registers every point in the circle. 4 times.

Eye exercises are concluded by opening eyes as wide as possible and then closing them tightly and blinking several times. This is done two to three times to activate the tear glands and to moisten the eyes. Then massage the eyes by gentle movements resembling the brushing of eyebrows with the thumb and index finger; then place hands in an attitude of prayer, with fingertips touching the point in the middle of the brows. Palms are parted with index fingers gently brushing under the eyes. Both of these movements are almost symbolic. You hardly touch your skin, but you are aware of the life force directed from the fingertips into your eyes.

Then place fingertips on top of eyes with thumbs underneath, forming a sort of five-digit cup with your hands. Deeply breathing in and out, form an image of bathing the eyes in rays of pranic energy emanating from the fingertips. The concluding practice is to vigorously rub the palms together until the sensation of heat develops in the palms, and then lightly cover both eyes with the cupped palms, enjoying the sensation of pleasant warmth. This technique is known as bathing the eyes in pranic energy.

The eyes always seem to be affected by a tired and rundown body condition. People in this condition often complain that they can't read small print, that they develop double vision, can't see objects distinctly and sharply. Yet two or three good nights of sleep and proper nourishment, rich with necessary vitamins, can restore or correct this condition completely. In my casebook there are testimonies of many people who improved their sight considerably with the improvement of their general health. On a number of occasions, people even in advanced years improved their eyesight enough so that they became capable of reading without glasses again and could dispense with them. One of my students experienced this phenomenon at the age of eighty-one. She claimed that she could read the telephone book again without eyeglasses for the first time in twenty years.

I would also like to make a comment about sunglasses. Dark sunglasses were practically unknown only fifty years ago. Now there are people who wear them literally all their waking hours, indoors and outdoors, in sunless weather and unwarranted circumstances. Many eye specialists are condemning this habit of overwearing sunglasses as generally harmful for the eyes. Of course, in bright snow while skiing or on a sunny beach, sunglasses are helpful, but people shouldn't wear them unnecessarily because they deny the eyes their natural amount of light and air.

In India, sunning of the eyes described in chapter 6 on energy from the elements is widely used as a means of restoring eyesight. Also recommended is the method of washing the eyes with tears, mentioned as one of the seven purifying processes in chapter 14 on rebirth.

Care of the Teeth, Hair, and Scalp

Care of the teeth should include regular and careful cleaning, of course, as well as massage of the gums by brushing and rubbing with the index finger and thumb. People with false teeth should be fastidious in hygiene. In addition, one's diet should include the kinds of food recommended in chapter 7 on diet: an abundance of raw fruits and vegetables and wholegrain bread, the chewing of which massages the gums.[1] A diet of soft, mushy foods will contribute to deterioration of facial muscles, teeth, and gums. Tooth problems are now studied the world over. It has been proved that in parts of the world where natural foods are eaten, teeth are far better than those in "civilized" countries where commercial foods predominate.

There are many exercises that benefit the teeth and gums. All the techniques involving the chin lock are important for blood circulation to the area of the mouth. The following are especially recommended: half shoulder stand, shoulder stand, triangular pose, cobra pose with the chin pressed in. Neck exercises described in this chapter are also beneficial for the teeth.

At a convention of dentists some years ago it was reported that the best teeth per capita of population were found in Bulgaria. Some dentists attributed this phenomenon to Bulgarian bread, which was very dense and required lots of chewing. It not only massages teeth and

---

1. The American habit of chewing gum may reflect an unconscious desire to exercise the teeth and gums. It definitely increases the flow of blood to the roots of the teeth.

gums, causing an extra flow of blood to the roots of the teeth, but it also serves as a good cleanser. I had the experience of meeting some Bulgarians well into their sixties and seventies who had never been to a dentist and who still had full sets of teeth. They claimed they had never used a toothbrush.

The Indian people are also famous for excellent teeth, but they are very particular about cleaning their teeth after each meal by chewing certain twigs which splinter on impact and remove particles of food from between the teeth.

In the yogic tradition, care of the teeth includes regular examination of your own mouth as well as cleaning of the teeth after each meal. In the mornings, gums are massaged with the fingers, gently but firmly squeezing and pulling gums on the upper jaw down (as if milking them), while gums of the lower jaw are massaged upward. This tradition is concerned with keeping the gums healthy and preventing them from receding and exposing the neck of the tooth, which is quite vulnerable to decay and infection. To whiten teeth you can use lemon juice once a week—enough to dip a toothbrush into is squeezed into the palm, and the teeth are brushed vigorously. One has to make a point of rinsing the mouth well several times with water afterward because lemon juice, due to its acidity, can contribute to the deterioration of the enamel if not removed. In the East, chalk, soda, or ashes are used in the place of toothpaste.

Traveling through India, on many occasions I met people with hair six to seven feet long. These were men belonging to a particular sect that specialized in growing very long hair. Their hair was usually plaited and arranged elaborately in garlands which rested on their shoulders; sometimes it was carried in a basket in front of the body. I spoke to these people, trying to find the secret of their achievement.

"We talk to our hair daily," said one. "We encourage it to grow. We do it regularly, and the hair starts to obey our commands." He also passed on to me another secret: Regular teasing with the tip of the tongue to the soft palate produces extensive saliva which is then swallowed; this is supposed to be very beneficial for the growth of hair.[2]

Apart from unorthodox ways to grow hair, massage of the scalp with the fingertips is highly recommended. Begin at the sides of the scalp: Vigorously move fingertips up and down, causing the scalp to move half a dozen times. Then change the position of the fingers to move the top part of the scalp vigorously. Change the position of the fingertips again and again until a sensation of pleasant warmth is achieved, indicating increased circulation in the area. This massage helps to prevent baldness and to grow stronger and healthier hair.

Regularity of these practices is the insurance for success. Scalp massage as well as facial exercises have to be performed once or even twice daily.

2. In the tradition of Chinese yoga, extensive salivation is achieved by champing the teeth thirty-six times and rolling the tongue (the "red dragon") for the same amount of time.

10

Rejuvenation by Sleep

Oh, gentle sleep! Nature's soft nurse. . . .
—Shakespeare

Shakespeare recognized the remarkable recuperative, curative, and invigorating properties of sleep. To him, sleeplessness was one of the greatest curses of man; it put one out of harmony with nature, ruining both body and mind.

Fifteen hundred years before Shakespeare, in ancient Greece, sick people were brought to the temple of Morpheus, the god of dreams, and left there overnight to recuperate. In the tradition of Taoist yoga, rejuvenation by sleep is one of the eighty rejuvenating techniques.

While in China I heard a legend about a Chinese emperor who was told by a fortune-teller that he would die in his sleep, so he vowed that he would not sleep anymore. Being a man with imagination, he devised a foolproof method to prevent him from falling asleep. He sat in a comfortable thronelike chair which allowed some amount of relaxation. He held in his right hand a heavy brass ball. Directly beneath it was a large brass basin.

Every time he started dozing, his fingers became relaxed and the brass ball fell with a tremendous noise into the basin, forcing him awake again. Within two months, the legend says, he went completely insane but cleverly concealed it from the court. At the beginning of the third month he fell on his own dagger to prove that he wouldn't die in his sleep.

Some animals will die by denial of sleep for a period as short as four days. It is now common knowledge that for normal growth and development of any living species, sleep is of great importance.

Modern scientific research into the phenomenon of sleep confirms many ancient ideas regarding the importance of sleep to health. As I mentioned earlier, a group of American researchers suggested that if people could be taught how to hibernate, their life expectancy could be doubled. Research into sleep goes on in practically every European country, as well as in America and Canada. It has been proved without any doubt that the source of some physical as well as mental maladies is a deficiency of sleep. When we lose sleep, mental and physical fatigue accumulate and can lead to the breakdown of even the strongest constitution.

One doctor put the problem graphically: We all have long lists of unpaid debts to the sleeping bank. If we do not pay them, we invite disaster.

Recently in Western Germany some tired executives chose to spend their annual holidays not in Cannes or Spain, but in a hospital engaged in marathon sleep, lasting up to two weeks. They emerged younger, healthier, and, in some cases, literally rejuvenated by this therapy. Other experiments have indicated that even one hour's extra sleep per night (comparing subjects who sleep seven hours with those who sleep eight) considerably reduces tension, fatigue, and nervous apprehension.

In many hospitals the importance of good sleep is recognized; patients are not wakened in the early morning hours for sponging and feeding, but instead are left undisturbed late into the morning hours. Sleep therapy proved especially important to children and elderly people, whose recuperative powers were greatly aided by it. Sleep therapists reported, "The period of time required to cure patients had been reduced 27 percent at one hospital; the death rate had been halved."

The first doctor in the Western world, Hippocrates, said that there are perhaps no better medicines than rest, sleep, and fasting. He himself was a good example of this teaching—he lived to be 106 years old. We spend about one-third of our lives in sleep or attempts to sleep, yet we too often take for granted that this important aspect of our lives will just take care of itself or that there is nothing we can do to improve it. Improving the quality of sleep is a great step toward conquering the ravages of time. To demonstrate this to yourself, try looking closely at yourself in a mirror after a restless night and compare that to the way your face looks after a good night of sleep. The effect of sleep on the eyes, on wrinkles, and on vitality is remarkable.

Chinese yoga includes the "art of big sleep," one of the techniques for improving the quality of life and increasing longevity. In "big sleep" the position of the bed is important. One should sleep with the head to the north and feet to the south in order not to disturb the magnetic field within the body. Apparently it was known to the ancients that the earth possesses its own magnetic field and that to put the body against the magnetic field of nature during sleep can be very disturbing to sleep. Many people would not register such a subtle effect as magnetic field interference, but some individuals are sensitive enough to be disturbed. In my casebook there are instances wherein people with a history of years of bad sleep improved their sleep dramatically the night the position of the bed was altered north to south.

The art of big sleep has a number of rules, starting with not eating any food after sunset. This is, of course, a stringent requirement that can be modified, if necessary, to not eating too much. It is common knowledge that one should not expect a long and invigorating sleep on going to bed with a full stomach of undigested food or after eating spices and salty food that make one thirsty. Warm water with honey will satisfy late evening "hunger" and is quickly digested.

The most important component of perfect sleep is physical and mental relaxation aided by full abdominal breathing. So many people complain that they feel tired early in the morning. One middle-aged student of mine told me a story that sounded absurd to me but which he was very serious about: He was so exhausted after a night of "sleep" that upon awakening he had to rest in his bed for another two hours before actually getting up and starting his work. This problem definitely points to shallow breathing during the night, wherein the bloodstream is not sufficiently oxygenated, resulting in the sensation of lassitude.

The essence of the art of sleep is the ability to breathe the deep abdominal breath in four major sleeping positions: on the right side, on the left side, on the back, and on the stomach. When this ability becomes a natural and unconscious act, a considerable amount of extra oxygen purifies the bloodstream. Abdominal breathing should be practiced in all four positions until the ability to breathe deeply in any position can be carried into sleep. Concentration on breathing is far better than counting sheep and will lead to healthy and natural sleep in a very short time, as rhythmical breath greatly helps to achieve perfect relaxation.

I was also taught that one should go to bed early, since the hours before midnight are the best hours of deep and undisturbed sleep. In the ashram where I learned the art of deep sleep, there was a rule to go to bed with the sunset and get up with sunrise. Recent studies of human cycles, as well as observation of the habits of healthy children who fall asleep long before midnight, indicate that there is much merit to the sunset-sunrise rule for sleeping. Perhaps for thousands of years we have been used to this particular bodily rhythm; only lately has man in urban societies interfered with it by staying up late with artificial lights and sleeping late into the day. Going to bed with sunset and getting up with sunrise may be unfeasible in an urban society, but at least we can train ourselves to go to bed early twice a week—on Wednesday night (the middle) not later than 9:00 P.M., as well as on Sunday night to start the new week well rested.

The mattress should be reasonably hard, without the sags that cause pressure on the spine, resulting in backache in the morning or even permanent injury to the spinal column. Pillows should be thin, and when you turn on the stomach, they should be pushed aside altogether, allowing the body to lie as flat as possible.

Another thing I learned in the ashram, which no doubt improved the quality of my sleep, was to wash my nasal passages regularly with warm, salted water, not only in the morning as a part of the seven purifying processes, but before retiring as well. During the hours of sleep, this procedure makes breathing much easier, eliminating "nightingales in the noses"—disturbing wheezing noises made during breathing, which in many cases could be the cause of insomnia.

It is a common thing in our society that marriage partners share the same bed, and in most cases the female partner suffers the disturbance of snoring. I have heard many complaints from women who are unable to sleep because of the snoring of their husbands. Although some women snore, it is more a male problem than a female one. Snoring occurs while sleeping on the back, when the muscles of the lower jaw relax and one breathes through the mouth, causing the soft palate to vibrate. In olden times, people were advised to wear chin straps to cure this problem, but of course that is not necessary if you train yourself in the art of nostril breathing and if your nasal passages are free from obstruction.

The marriage bed is often not wide enough, restricting natural movements of the partners during the night, which leads to disturbed sleep. Of course, the ideal sleep occurs while in your own bed, especially after the age of fifty when the capacity to sleep has declined.

An anecdote about marital sleeping habits professes that in your twenties it is so pleasant to sleep in each other's arms; in your forties you may still share the same bed with some pleasure; in your fifties you must graduate to separate beds in order to sleep well; and in your seventies you depart to different rooms. There is some merit to this guideline.

Another suggestion for better sleep is to be sure that you have quiet in your sleeping chambers. It is not uniform and continuous noises like the ticking of a clock that keep people awake, but rather the erratic and sudden loud noises of traffic, machinery, and the like. In cases when these noises are unavoidable, earplugs are recommended to filter a certain amount of the noise.

Millions of people throughout the world know unconsciously about the recuperative powers of sleep. They go to bed when they feel "out of sorts." It is not unusual in cases of mental stress for people to escape into sleep and wake up refreshed and cured, with their mental problems sorted out by the computer of unconsciousness.

There is an ancient Russian proverb, "Morning is wiser than evening," which suggests that a mind freshened by a night of good sleep functions better and more clearly than a fatigued mind.

Now we know more about sleep than perhaps at any time in human history. We know that the deepest sleep is a dreamless one, whereas sleep with dreams is light, when the unconscious tries to communicate with the conscious mind through dream symbols. The unconscious mind knows more about our health than the conscious mind. Many doctors, in cases of difficult diagnoses, discuss dreams with their patients, trying to find the source of a malady and its cure. Dreams related to one's health should be carefully analyzed, either by intensive self-study supported by related information from psychological studies or by therapy.

As I mentioned in the beginning of the discussion of sleep, scientists think that hibernation could double the life expectancy. Amazingly enough, the ancient yogis knew this. One of my Indian teachers demonstrated a famous *kechari mudra*, a highly advanced technique to prolong the life span. In the *kechari mudra*, the tongue is lengthened by the process of "milking," or pulling on, the tongue with the fingers for a period of many weeks. Some of the experts eventually were capable of touching the bridges of their noses with their tongues. Before going to bed at night, the lengthened tongue was rolled backward, closing the glottis. This produces a state greatly resembling hibernation: Respiration and metabolism are slowed considerably; the blood pressure and rate of heartbeat are reduced. In this state, according to the belief, the body does not age. A master of the *kechari mudra* spends every second night in this attitude, thus prolonging his life span.

The yogi who demonstrated this technique to me was

eighty-four years old but looked a youthful fifty. I will never forget my amazement when, looking into his mouth to observe the correct procedure for this *mudra,* I saw a full set of teeth which, though yellow, were perfectly intact. As I questioned him in more detail, he told me that the *kechari mudra* is extremely dangerous because of the possibility of choking yourself with your own tongue. It can be learned only under the close and continuous supervision of an expert.

Many older people develop an almost paranoid fear of sleep because they are frightened of dying in their sleep. Mark Twain reflected this fear when he advocated, "Never go to bed; too many people die there." Among older people, there is a real fear of even a temporary loss of consciousness when death might suddenly creep up on one.

We should train ourselves to love and to welcome sleep, which is not only a restorer of vital forces, but from a metaphysical point of view, an adventure into a different and unknown realm. A poet (I. Odoyevtseva), in a delightful poem about sleep, wrote, "I enjoy my life equally in a conscious state and in my sleep." I am perfectly certain that mastery of the art of perfect sleep could increase the life span by fifteen to twenty years.

11

Rejuvenation by Love

An ancient Indian legend tells of a prince who met a maiden with the body of a goddess and the languid and longing eyes of a gazelle in springtime. He told her, "I know why you are wearing this black sari embroidered in gold—because in a primeval forest you were a tigress and I was a tiger. My soul recognizes your soul." Afterward, in competition with the nobles of the court, the prince shot an arrow seven miles, felled a tree with one stroke of his sword, and jumped over a wide gorge on his stallion. The prince's extraordinary accomplishments were, of course, inspired by having found his beloved. When two true lovers meet—when soul recognizes soul—the strength of the partners multiplies severalfold. Nothing, then, is impossible to achieve.

According to the ancient tradition, during the golden age of humanity, there was a state of unity between male and female when they truly were one entity. People were beautiful androgynes—wise, serene, perfectly contented. An envious spirit dissected them into halves and scattered these halves all over the world. Since then, men and women have searched for their "other halves," darkly confused, rarely discovering their true counterparts.

The roots of both legends are in the Shiva-Shakti principle of the Tantric yoga tradition: Man is Shiva, creator; woman is Shakti, energy which makes creation possible. Together they make up the world.

The ancients recognized the rejuvenating properties of love; that is why rituals for lovemaking were incorporated into the Tantric tradition. Philosophically, the roots of love are in immortality. Love represents the procreation of new life, as well as psychic reintegration through the union of opposites.

Anyone who has truly been in love knows that it is the most wonderful experience of a lifetime. It suffuses one's being on all levels, so much so that lovers often become spontaneously engaged in a kind of courtly love meditation in which the image of the beloved is carried continuously in the mind of the lover, illuminating the soul and creating an atmosphere of eternal spring.

Scientific reports are contradicting the old fallacy that too much sexual intercourse ages a person; on the contrary, it helps to keep one young. There is no doubt of the rejuvenating effect of falling in love. Numerous instances have been recorded of the vanishing of signs of aging as a result of falling in love: Wrinkles, age spots, poor posture, brittleness disappear as we move with greater vitality and grace, see life with greater hope and expectation, and generally behave in a much younger way. I recently heard the testimony of a psychiatrist that a woman in her fifties who fell in love for the first time grew at least twenty years younger, even to such an extent that her menstrual cycle came back to her on a regular basis. Rejuvenation by love has been mentioned in Chinese, Indian, Japanese, and Persian literary traditions. We also read about it in the Bible, where Solomon's "Song of Songs" is an ode to love.

Our Western tradition has extolled courtly or romantic love in its poetry, drama, and novels, as well as in most other forms of artistic expression. Inevitably in these representations the lovers expect their intensity of feeling to last "forever after." Yet if we study the literature that peeks into married life, we always get the impression that romance has vanished while dreariness, bitterness, resentment, boredom, and sometimes violence have taken over the domestic scene.

When we first fall in love we have the eyes of a prince looking at a princess, a worthy and enchanting consort. We are inspired by a pleasing encounter to build with our imaginations a concept of a relationship that befits a god and a goddess. Perhaps the disappointments of married life come from a failure of imagination by both partners. It is difficult to sustain awareness of the god in oneself and the goddess in one's partner without ritual support. That is why the Tantric ritual of *maithuna* can be helpful.

To maintain interest in a relationship, the sex act, which in the West is often identified with love, must be elevated from the purely physical, sometimes animallike level onto a higher plane. Then sex becomes a divine and deeply mystical act, an important aspect of spiritual growth, exemplified in the practice of *maithuna*. When sex is brought to this level, the entire psyche of the partners is readjusted; indeed, one's whole life and environment are transformed.

My purpose here is not to write a full treatise on Tantric yoga, which I explored at some length in an earlier book, *Sex and Yoga,* but to introduce the reader to the idea that the sex act can become a powerful rejuvenating medium for those who are prepared to open their minds to love's dark and beautiful, mystical side. Married couples, using the principles and techniques of ancient Tantric tradition, can put back a flame into their dwindling or stale relationship and find a source of new and subtle pleasure in the love act as well as in the entire man-woman concept of togetherness.

The traditional *maithuna,* or sexual union of the Tantric practices, holds the secret to the spiritual readjustment of the partners. In this ritual the woman is elevated into the status of a goddess, and her Shakti, or energy power, is recognized by her partner; in turn, he impersonates for her the creator Shiva. Through these recognitions, both move onto a much higher plane of consciousness where gentleness substitutes for roughness, adoration and desire for force of habit, a set of new values for a mundane attitude toward everyday life. *Maithuna,* if performed properly, will leave a lasting effect on the psyche of both partners. The memories of this ritual will remain to ward off unkindness, mistrust, or boredom.

Under these circumstances, the sexual union itself is a magical act, full of rejuvenating potential. The sexual union becomes no longer a casual, offhand conjugal rite experienced by the husband as mere relief from sexual pressure or by the wife as one more duty to be gotten out of the way, but a beautiful mystery that both partners approach with desire and anticipation.

The ritual of *maithuna* is traditionally performed on the fifth day after cessation of menstruation or, in the case of a woman whose menstrual experience is past, on the fifth day of each month. The first *maithuna* should be performed after at least two weeks of abstinence from sexual intercourse to intensify the pleasure of it; thereafter, it can be practiced when desired.

There are many varieties of *maithuna* in the Tantric tradition, some of which stress the retention of seminal energy during the actual coitus, some allowing the movement of semen into the vagina but including a very complex and extremely difficult act of drawing this flow back into the penis (believed to be achieved by extraordinary mastery over involuntary muscles which normally cannot be controlled). In the Western world, for the Western householder, these techniques are undesirable and even dangerous. In describing the sexual union below, I am showing the middle way for married householders, which has all the qualities of the traditional *maithuna* and leads partners onto a higher plane of consciousness.

In a way, *maithuna* is a very elaborate courtship ritual; Every detail of attire, food, drink, scent, and even light has a specified part to play. Prior to union, both partners bathe. The woman scents her body with perfumed oil. She wears a loose red gown (hibiscus or cardinal red is a color associated with passion); her partner is dressed in white (to symbolize purity). She is dressed to evoke his passion; he is dressed to indicate the purity of his intentions.

The room where *maithuna* is performed should be aesthetically pleasing, warm, and illuminated by a single source of light (lantern or lamp) with a violet cover. In the Tantric tradition, violet stimulates sexual desire more than any other color, even red. During the actual practice of *maithuna*, the beam of light should be adjusted to fall directly on the sexual features of the female body (not for the partner's benefit so much as for the woman's—tradition teaches that this violet light has a powerful stimulating effect on the sex chakra in the female).

The room should contain a bed that is wide and firm and a table for food and drink in close proximity to the bed. Traditionally, the food is of four kinds, symbolizing the elements: earth (bread), air (meat), water (fish), and fire (wine). The female partner enters the room first and waits for the male. She is beautifully attired and full of anticipation. Then the male partner enters and sits with her upon the bed, whereupon the feast begins.

The feast is not designed to appease hunger; it is a

ritual ceremony pregnant with symbolic meaning. The wine is opened and the bouquet inhaled by the male through the left nostril, with exhalation through the right. This act symbolizes the purification of the *nadis,* or nervous-psychic channels, of the male partner. Only three small glasses of wine are consumed by each partner during the ritual, and only a small amount of each kind of food is taken. By eating and drinking these foods, the partners are acknowledging the role of these represented elements in their lives and are bringing themselves into harmony with them.

It is always strongly advocated that neither of the partners should be overfull or even slightly intoxicated at the end of the feast. A small amount of water with lemon juice is consumed to purify the mouth at the end of the feast. The partners offer each other a cardamom seed in very much the same way as the ritual exchange of wedding rings. They chew small portions of the seeds (the cardamom seed is enclosed in a husk or shell and represents the soul encased in the sheath of the body). Partners then disrobe and lie down on the bed, transformed by their anticipation of what is to happen into "beautiful, wise, and serene gods."

Foreplay is carried out in a traditional manner before consummation. The male partner touches his Shakti very gently on the forehead, lips, both nipples, and then he places his hand lightly on her "mount of Venus," where the light falls. She responds by touching his navel, caressing his stomach, then taking his penis in her right hand. Though both are sexually aroused at this stage, both remain on a spiritually high level of consciousness—he visualizing her as a goddess of love, she seeing him as the creator Shiva.

Lying on her back, the female partner draws her knees up as the male on his left side moves his upper torso away from her, bringing his penis into close contact with the lips of her vagina. He places his right leg between her thighs and inserts his penis halfway. For the next half hour the two partners lie in silence and stillness, meditating upon the Shiva-Shakti union on various levels of being. Passionate whispers are replaced by the most noble and gentle medium of thoughts on the highest level. They breathe rhythmically. The male should lie within a good view of his beloved. In this manner, the desire slowly mounts in both bodies. Finally, there is a spasmodic contraction of the vagina of Shakti which literally draws the penis full-length into her body, squeezing it with the muscles of her vagina and bringing both to a point of ecstatic joy in orgasm, experienced by both partners with the same intensity and at exactly the same time.

The next few minutes are filled with supreme joy. The physical body is relieved of sexual desire, but *maithuna* continues on a higher plane toward the ultimate goal of illumination or supreme bliss, a unification of the individual spirit with the spirit of the universe. In the yogic tradition, it is believed that a state of *samadhi* is achieved at this moment; through physical union, both partners are completely reintegrated personally and also brought into unity with the cosmos, experiencing a state of cosmic consciousness. It is at this moment of the union of opposites that one experiences the feeling of rejuvenation.

12

Mental Training

Yoga is a philosophy of complete development in which mental, physical, and spiritual potentialities are cultivated and brought into the highest possible state of attainment and balance. We see in the lotus posture of yoga a triangle which represents among other things the three facets of human growth. As I indicated earlier, the triangle symbolized much the same in ancient Greece. In preceding chapters I have described some of the techniques for building a physical foundation for renewal and growth. Now I would like to focus on the role of mental training in health and long life.

We have already discussed the need to reprogram our psyches so that we can see the rich potentiality for continuing mental education and spiritual growth and for maintaining bodily grace, suppleness, beauty, and strength as we mature. In this chapter we will be concerned with exercises that can help us sharpen our mental faculties.

Early in the book I described some of the symptoms of aging as they are reflected in the decline of mental powers: failing memory, the inability to concentrate, vulnerability to upsurges of the unconscious in which we become preoccupied with the past. In addition to these failing powers, people are often plagued with regrets that they did not develop more of their personality potentials.

We know that exercise is largely responsible for the body's good condition, yet it often comes as a surprise to realize that exercise of a different kind determines one's good mental condition. Mental powers, if not exercised, atrophy just as muscles of the body atrophy if not used. For example, members of the younger generation who have grown up watching too much television may have sacrificed much of their ability to imagize. Constant bombardment from without deprives us of the opportunity to create our own images—an opportunity that is present in reading and even listening to the radio, two pastimes that have been usurped by television for many people.

Similarly, the inability to concentrate is a problem among the young as well as the old. Sensory overload leads to apathetic mental functioning. Further, we live in a society that demands specialization; to survive economically, we mold ourselves into specialists, thus fragmenting the natural human impulse toward diverse and rounded growth.

This tendency toward specialization has the advantage of producing virtual geniuses within a limited sphere. For instance, we in the Western world have attained great heights in the use of our rational powers. The gains that have been made in science and technology have given tremendous prestige to rationalism in the West. Nevertheless, it is to some extent our misfortune that we have specialized in such a way because we have sadly neglected such powers as imagination and intuition. Of course, there have been geniuses of imagination and intuition in our culture, but these faculties are all too often considered the province of eccentrics. Properly, they are the province of everyone. Fragmentation can be found in our attitude toward mathematics, language, music, and art. We often hear someone say, "He has a mathematical mind," or "She has a propensity for language," or "He is so fortunate to have musical or artistic talent." The ability to be creative in these spheres is a potential in all of us, but the potentials will remain only latent if the opportunity for their development does not occur or if we become prejudiced against these interests because we see them as rare abilities given only to a few.

Some branches of yoga philosophy such as Raja or Kundalini yoga teach that we use only a negligible part of our mental powers—maybe as little as one-tenth; modern scientists suggest the same. We all believe that in the natural evolution of mankind these powers will be developed, yet we tend to think that it may take thousands of years. Nevertheless, there are some exciting research results on the human brain now being published that offer us new perspectives and new hopes that some advancement may be made in our lifetime.

Researchers have shown that the brain apparently has two hemispheres of operation: The left lobe seems to control the linear thought processes that pertain to language and mathematics; the right lobe governs processes in which clusters and constellations are important, such as can be found in image making, musical activity, and intuitive response. Our emphasis on rational and linear thought suggests that we in the West have developed the left hemisphere of the brain but have neglected the right. In our time, the field of holistic psychology has developed out of a need to bring the two hemispheres into balance—to make a wholeness of ourselves. Perhaps our current interest in Eastern thought and occult practices arises out of a need to set right the imbalance of our tendency for the past few centuries to operate only in the sphere of the left brain.

Parapsychology is one among many new and fertile

fields of growth in thought. Just what are we capable of mentally? Psychokinesis (influence of mind over matter)? Telepathy? Astral travel? We don't know exactly because we don't have enough results from scientifically controlled experiments. But we have learned enough to be open and receptive to the vast possibilities of achievement in these areas. Surely this century has taught us that science fiction may quickly become fact. The early stories by Jules Verne about submarines and flying machines were just as strange to his first readers as astral projection and psychokinesis are to us. Yet submarines and airplanes are commonplace now. A few years hence, mental telepathy and levitation may be commonplace.

In two countries—Russia and Japan—these latent potentialities of the human mind are being taken quite seriously on a nationwide scale, just as in America they are coming under the aegis of scientific experimentation at such places as Duke University, the University of Virginia, and the Menninger Clinic.

I am making all these speculations to establish a context for the yoga tradition of mental training. In the yoga tradition, these mental powers are referred to as *sidhas.* A description of some of them is more fascinating than any science fiction story. The *sidhas* include the ability to become lighter than air, to become invisible, to project one's "astral self" with the speed of thought to any part of the world, and to cause objects to materialize out of thin air. Impossible? Well, don't discount our current science fictions as harbingers of actual accomplishments on the part of humankind.

Nevertheless, our purpose here is not to teach people how to fly or to become invisible, but rather to develop powers important in our day-to-day lives which contribute to our total growth, including radiant health and longevity. Whether we develop these vaster powers of the

mind which seem so out of reach is not particularly important to our program. But it is important that we rouse
ourselves to the greater mental challenges that we often
relegate to the "outstanding" members of our culture,
thinking that we ourselves are not capable of great
achievement. These challenges are ever present to all
of us. Our task is to meet them.

One of the richest opportunities of maturity is to explore dormant personality potentials. The casebooks of
Jungian psychologists, for instance, are filled with examples of people in their middle and late years who discovered latent artistic abilities as they became interested
in expressing their experiences of personal growth.

Concentration, imagination, and willpower can be
strengthened and increased by the willing and dedicated
person. It is perhaps true that some people have more
innate drive to develop these powers than others. Even
so, we acknowledge the truth in the cliché that behind
every great work is a moment of inspiration and tons
of perspiration and that "talent" is 10 percent genius
and 90 percent hard work.

This brings me to a subject that I approach with some
trepidation because it has become a cliché in American
life through the enormous popular success of Norman
Vincent Peale's book *The Power of Positive Thinking*.
In yoga training one is taught to cultivate the ability to
think positively; it is an essential skill in developing the
powers of the mind. An important distinction should be
made between shallow credulity or gullibility in the face
of life's experience, and the more profound determination to turn unfortunate or unpleasant experience into a
satisfying meaningfulness. In this form of mental training
one tries to see all things whole: Whatever may seem
at the moment to yield only negative results usually, when
placed in perspective, will yield at least a germ of positive

result. And that germ can be the basis of a new and creative adventure.

We forget sometimes that what we are and what we do is largely determined by what we think. Poor mental health is usually treated by reeducation of the patient's thoughts and his self-image. Although not so widely recognized, the same is true of physical health: In a way, it is a matter of reeducation.

Some doctors today think that not less than 75 percent of all maladies begin in the mind. Other doctors are more conservative, but few medical practitioners doubt anymore that many diseases have a psychosomatic origin. The old country doctors were acknowledging that fact when they prescribed "little pink pills" for a wide variety of maladies, diagnosed as much by the doctor's hunch about the patient's mental state as by any other symptoms. The widespread use of the placebo demonstrates that the body can and does heal itself; the doctor may help, of course, and drugs may be useful, but one's own body must take the initiative for any healing to occur.

I believe, as ancient yoga sages have taught, that we can determine our state of health by the power of positive thinking. The effect of our thinking upon our bodies is so profound that we can think "young" and instantly feel better and more energetic; we can think "thin" and more easily reduce excess weight. We can think "healthy" and develop the sensation of physical well-being.

If you find yourself easily frustrated or inclined toward a morose view of life, one of your first tasks should be to train yourself to search for meaning and positive potential in your circumstances. This searching can lead you into profound meditations (the subsequent chapter on meditation, particularly the exercise of sorting thoughts and attitudes, may be helpful).

Try reeducating your attitudes by simple procedures:

Approach unpleasant tasks and dreaded conversations with a positive expectation; rouse yourself to the mental challenge to create positive images of yourself, your circumstances, your expectations.

As we reach middle age, we tend to think of our mental and physical habits as fixed. We grow comfortable with our patterns of behavior, even though they may have caused us to fall far short of our youthful goals. We may still yearn to accomplish great works outwardly or inwardly but feel that our chance to do so has passed. It is unfortunate that many of us give in easily to comfort or despair. Why settle for second- or third-rate expression of our infinitely rich potentials? Even though you may believe in reincarnation, the prospects of this life are still provocative, and they don't diminish after age forty or fifty or sixty.

The exercises below are designed to sharpen mental faculties where they are already in use, and to arouse latent or dormant mental faculties, partly because their use is satisfying in itself and partly because we need sharp mental faculties to aid in our physical and spiritual rejuvenation. In the final section I present some of the possibilities for achieving greater mental control over our state of health by the use of self-hypnosis.

Exercises to Develop Concentration

Do not desire anything too strongly—it may come to you.
—Spanish proverb

The proverb attests to the cultural universality of a seemingly magical power in concentration, or focusing one's attention supremely on a goal. Concentration of one's attention does involve a wish or a desire—the desire to embrace single-mindedly one objective and to exclude any distraction that might interfere with one's aim, whether momentary or long-range.

Eastern metaphysical traditions often assert that wish is the most powerful influence in the world—that with a conscious wish, anything can be attained. In Tibetan yoga, concentration has the attribute of magic. It is considered the skill or force behind all endeavors. The apparent "magic" involved in concentration can be traced to our difficulty in attending to a goal. To attend means to work lovingly toward a cause or aim. Yet we are so vulnerable to distraction!

The degree of our concentration makes all the difference toward the success or failure of anything we try to do, whether cooking, writing, playing chess, working mathematical problems, or engaging in sports. Athletes probably know better than anyone else how important concentration is to excellence in performance. It is fitting, I think, to consider the importance of concentration in our program of rejuvenation.

Patanjali, in his third book of *sutras,* describes concentration as a "binding of the perceiving consciousness to a certain region." Concentration is one-pointedness of the mind, the ability to focus attention on a problem, idea, or thought. In a similar vein, Sir Isaac Newton asserted that he made his great discoveries by "intending his mind on them." Concentration can be developed by a series of exercises which are united by one principle: directing the beam of the perceiving consciousness to the object of concentration.

EXERCISE 1: Concentration on a Black Spot

Seated in a cross-legged position, breathing deeply and rhythmically, concentrate your gaze on a small black spot painted on a piece of white paper. Be sure that not just the sight but the mind is engaged in this effort to concentrate entirely on the black spot. If the mind wanders, bring it back again and again, trying to lengthen the time of its focus on the spot. Start with a few minutes in the beginning; gradually try to concentrate for at least 15 minutes without letting the mind wander about. This exercise is particularly good at helping you to train yourself to exclude distractions.

EXERCISE 2: Concentration on a Candle Flame
Perform the same exercise as above, this time using a candle flame instead of a black spot. This exercise is usually done in a darkened room. Take care not to strain your eyes.

EXERCISE 3: Concentration on the Point Between the
Eyebrows
Posture and breathing are the same as above. Close your eyes. Roll your eyes up and concentrate your mind on the point between the eyebrows. Lengthen the time of concentration as before.

EXERCISE 4: Concentration on the Tip of the Nose
Posture and breathing are the same as above. Turn the eyes inward to focus on the tip of the nose. This exercise involves a certain amount of effort on the part of the semivoluntary muscles of the eyes as the eyeballs are turned toward each other. The position is retained for a few moments, gradually extending the duration of the gaze but again avoiding eye fatigue at all costs. Because this exercise breaks our normal way of focusing sight, it is conducive to altering one's state of consciousness.

EXERCISE 5: Concentration on Empty Space
Seated and breathing as above, eyes open, focus the gaze on empty space about 12 inches from the tip of the nose. Since there is no concrete point of fixation,

this exercise is more difficult than the others given before; it offers a greater challenge to retain one-pointedness of the mind.

EXERCISE 6: Concentration on Sound

The first exercise of concentration on sound should be to focus on the sound of incoming and outgoing breath. Recall the mantra of health in which the sound *so* is made for incoming breath and *hum* for outgoing breath. Concentrate on these sounds as you breathe, retaining focus for as long as possible. Then you can isolate other sounds for exercises in concentration.

EXERCISE 7: Concentration on Thought and Action

After these elementary exercises in concentration, you can begin to bring your power of concentration to bear on more complex problems of thought and action. For instance, you can pick out problem areas in your program for rejuvenation. If you are overweight, you can practice concentrating single-mindedly on weight loss; if you are stiff, you can practice concentrating on becoming more supple.

Posture and breathing are the same as above. Close your eyes. Concentrate on a single thought, such as *I am going to become thinner* or *I am going to become more supple*. Hold the thought in mind for as long as possible without distraction. When you emerge from such prolonged concentration, you will be more resolute about translating thought into action. You will be able to experience some of the "magic" of binding your attention to a goal.

Before embarking on any serious project you should concentrate on its aspects until you have clearly in mind what you need to do and until you are inwardly fortified to do it. Remember that anything can be achieved by the power of the wish, provided your concentration supports the wish.

All these exercises in concentration lead to greater lucidity in sensory impressions as well as greater ability to influence one's state of consciousness. They lead directly to the exercises in imagination which follow and indirectly to the meditation practices given in chapter 13.

Exercises to Develop Imagination

Imagination is the power to create something out of nothing—nothing that is apparent, anyway. Within the mind is a corollary for all of our senses, so that we can speak of the mind's eye or the inner voice that we hear, not with our auditory sense, but with our imagination. We know how smell can evoke a long journey into the past because our mind has retained an image of a certain odor from many years ago. A girl reported to me that she tried for years to duplicate the taste of her grandmother's apple cake. No recipe was available; the grandmother had been dead for fifteen years. All the girl had was a vivid memory of a taste. When she finally hit on the right combination of butter, eggs, milk, sugar, and flour, poured the right number of thin layers and baked them, covered them with a sauce made from simmering dried apples and cinnamon, and tasted the result, she had a mystical experience of having made a bridge in time.

All poets, besides creating from their own imagination, draw heavily on their knowledge of images such as those we all have locked in our minds. Poems are replete with images of sight, sound, touch, smell, and taste. Through such images the poet engages his own imagination with that of the reader.

Basically, the power of imagination is the power to

imagize in concrete form what is not present, whether it be a simple image or a highly complex one—a single memory or a plan for a whole country's growth and development. Imagination is generally known to us as a power which can transform the world around us or create a new world within. It is a very important power in any creative work. Like concentration, this power can be strengthened and developed.

There are a number of exercises to develop the power of imagination. In concentration exercises, actual objects are usually used as a focus; in developing the imagination, those objects are replaced by images.

EXERCISE 1: Imaging Colors

Seated cross-legged, breathing deeply and rhythmically, close your eyes. Choose any favorite color of the spectrum, and use your entire concentration to visualize this color as clearly as possible without any mental interference. Retain the image for as long as possible. After working on your favorite color, pass from one to another of every color in the spectrum, trying to retain concentration on each color for as long as possible.

EXERCISE 2: Re-creating One's Surroundings

Seated cross-legged or relaxed in a comfortable armchair, one imagines a beautiful landscape or seascape in great detail. Then he imagines himself as a part of the landscape, taking it all in through his senses. Each detail should be savored.

In my casebook there is an incredible story in which one of my students acquired an actual sunburn while sunning in an imaginary landscape. Once, while conducting a seminar on meditation, I introduced an exercise to develop the power of concentration. I asked my students to sit cross-legged with eyes closed, breathing deeply and rhythmically. I suggested that they imagine themselves at a seashore on a beautiful, sunny summer day. I advised them to concentrate as much as they could on the sunshine touching their faces and bodies. After ten minutes of practice one of the students, a young girl, walked to the stage where I was seated and asked me to look at her face. Her face was definitely red, and there was a triangular patch of redness that followed the lines created by the neckline of her blouse. We all moved to a large mirror to view the phenomenon together. Everyone in the class was amazed. The girl told me that she terminated her exercise when she realized that if she continued for another few minutes she would actually develop a sunburn.

Obviously, this girl possessed a remarkable susceptibility to suggestion. Other reactions of the people in the class to my suggestion varied from no response whatever to the experience of pleasant warmth, which was predominant. That incident verified again for me that there is a strong relationship between mind and body because the physical change was produced in the skin of her body by thought alone. It seems only logical to assume that many reactions, positive or negative changes, can be evoked by the power of thinking.

Another student told me that the exercise of imagination saved his life. He was a Japanese prisoner of war in Burma, subjected to unbelievable hardships and trials in building the Burma Road. During the middle of the day there was a half-hour break when a little food was given out. He trained himself to chew every morsel thoroughly to extract all nutrition. Then he would lie down to relax in the shade of some bushes at the roadside. He would imagine himself back in his native Devonshire. He recalled in detail the garden of his cottage, the smell of flowering shrubbery and roses, the soft wind, the countryside. He told me that he perfected this exercise to such an extent that for fifteen minutes he was more in England than in Burma. He would come out of this imaginary trip to his homeland refreshed and invigorated physically and spiritually. He developed during these practices a powerful belief that he would survive, and he did.

Romain Gary, in *Roots of Heaven,* describes a similar story in which a man survives a concentration camp by imagining herds of elephants roaming freely over Africa. He survived to dedicate his life to saving the elephants from extinction.

EXERCISE 3: Screen of the Forehead

In this exercise, which is also used for meditative practices, after the cross-legged position and rhythmical breath have been established, look at your own forehead from inside the skull as if you are looking at a small screen. You can project various images onto the screen—whatever is particularly soothing to you: a beautiful medieval castle, or a lovely villa high up in the mountains, or an Oriental garden. These images can become amazingly real as the power of your imagination grows.

The exercises to develop the imagination are all fascinating and rewarding mental practices. One who has learned the power of imagination can never again be bored with himself or tormented by loneliness.

Exercises to Develop the Mind's Eye

Although the general public is not even aware of the existence of the mind's eye, it plays a very important role in yoga, as well as in the imaginative work of poets, writers, and artists of all cultures. There are similarities and differences between the mind's eye and the imagination. The mind's eye is a tool of the imagination. It is the visual aspect of imagination, particularly as it relates to one's past experiences. It is the ability to recreate an image, for example, of the house one lived in ten years ago or the face of a friend or relative one has not seen for a while. The mind's eye is identified by many investigators of higher aspects of yoga philosophy with the pineal gland, which in this tradition is considered a dormant organ of the higher faculties of human makeup.

Apart from the ability to recreate images and happenings of the past, the mind's eye has another faculty— the ability to see into one's body. A fully evolved yoga adept can see into his body as if he had acquired some kind of X-ray vision. A man engaged in mind research, and at one stage experimenting with LSD, told me that he had acquired this ability to see into his body. I do not intend here to speculate on the likelihood of acquiring X-ray vision, but in the context of yoga training, through the practice of the inverted gaze, a much better awareness of the inner life of the body can be acquired. We must keep in mind also that there is only a short distance from awareness to mastery over these functions.

EXERCISE 1: Re-creating an Object from a Distance
in Space
Sitting behind your breakfast table, have a good look at it, then walk into another room and try to describe what was on it, recreating it in detail by the power of the mind's eye.

EXERCISE 2: Traveling into the Past
Sitting in a cross-legged position, rhythmical breath established, imagine a beautiful scene from your past trav-

els—a place that impressed you. Travel to this place again and again in your exercise, trying to see it better and better with the mind's eye.

EXERCISE 3: Re-creating a House from Ten Years' Distance in Time

Think of a house you lived in ten years ago. Go through it with your mind's eye, room after room, trying to see it again. Remember colors, textures, and shapes, as if you were actually there again.

EXERCISE 4: Travel into Your Body

For this purpose, it is worthwhile to review human biology by looking at pictures of the interior of the body so that you can more accurately visualize what is happening as you exercise.

While deeply and rhythmically breathing, look with your mind's eye at your diaphragm. Try to gain awareness of its movement. Travel to the lower part of your lungs and again, using the mind's eye, become conscious of how they are filled up and emptied in the process of breathing.

Whenever you are exercising, try to visualize the effect of the exercise on your body's interior. For example, when you practice *nauli* or *uddiyan,* try to see with your mind's eye the effect of the massage on your vital organs. Become aware of your heart's pulsations by visualizing them as they occur. This awareness helps you to gain the capability of controlling the pulsations.

EXERCISE 5: Search for Tension

A typical exercise to develop the power of the mind's eye is a search for tension in the body. This exercise is usually performed as the second stage of the exercise of complete relaxation (see Index). After bringing the muscles into relaxation, the mind's eye turns inward and slowly travels over the body in an effort to recognize possible zones of tension. When a pocket of tension is discovered by this process, an additional effort of will is exerted to relax the tension.

EXERCISE 6: Limbering Up the Spine

In the limbering-up movement for the spinal column in chapter 8 on shaping the body, the student is trained to visualize his spine and the movement in every socket of his vertebrae.

EXERCISE 7: Breathing for Recharging the Body

In the exercise that involves breathing for recharging the body, the mind's eye plays an important part. The student visualizes the process: With the incoming breath he absorbs *prana* into his system and with outgoing breath he directs it to every cell of the body. He is trained to see with his mind's eye how he is directing energy to his solar plexus or to various vital organs of the body and nervous centers.

EXERCISE 8: Creating a Protective Aura

Another typical example of the use of the mind's eye is in the exercise of creating a protective aura. The student first imagines that with each exhalation he directs the life force through every pore of his skin, creating a protective cocoon around his body. Then he actually sees this aura with his mind's eye. In the Tibetan art of *dumo*, or creating psychic heat, the yogi dresses himself in the warm cloth of his breath, which is visible only to his mind's eye.

Metaphysical teachings attribute to the mind's eye many more properties, including the ability to see people's auras, chakras, or fields of energy, or to see the invisible world as a different dimension within our visible one. For our purposes, we can say that the use of the mind's eye in various exercises evokes in turn a constructive power of thinking. In meditative practices, the frequent use of the mind's eye eventually leads to greater self-realization.

Development of Willpower

Willpower is the greatest source of inner strength. In the Chinese tradition, inner strength is called "the sister of courage." The will can be defined as the ability to make decisions; inner strength is what makes possible accomplishment from these decisions. Like all other mental powers, the will can atrophy from want of use. Perhaps it is the most susceptible to atrophy of all our mental faculties.

Life gives us innumerable opportunities to exercise will. Many people are not conscious that they can exercise willpower and often opt for comfort, no matter what the challenge. They glide with the obvious and easy currents of life, relatively satisfied with whatever life sends their way. Gliding becomes a habit; willpower dissipates and may disappear. A person who is basically upright and wholesome may yet, because he has no willpower, fall prey to unsavory or unfortunate experiences in life.

Alcohol, for instance, prevents a complicated challenge to the will. One of the negative aspects of alcohol is its power to undermine and eventually destroy willpower.

The physical practices of yoga are not only challenging to the body; in many cases they are greater challenges to the willpower. The very effort of exercising requires an element of willpower; as we meet each day's—each moment's—challenge, not only does the body grow stronger but the willpower is exercised and strengthened as well.

You can begin to develop willpower in this way: Make an inner promise that you will try never again to choose the easy path. Avoid the temptation to give in to the old habits of behavior that are unsatisfactory to your best self. Begin with small things if necessary: Refuse to eat when you know only habit is calling. I know many people who have discovered that they are much happier not eating until past noon each day; others run to the kitchen at the first growl of an overfed and spoiled appetite, as if in fear that they will be devoured by it if they don't feed it. Refuse to be dominated by habits or appetites. Refuse to put off unpleasant but necessary confrontations or conversations. Thoreau has written an excellent essay on this subject in *Walden.* In the process of living, learn how to exercise your willpower. You will be rewarded by the wonderful feeling of victory over the weaknesses in yourself.

The development of the will naturally leads to the development of inner strength—a wonderful and noble quality of human makeup that is immediately recognizable in the people who have it. It is a positive aspect of the spiritually active person, implying not brute force but the strength of intelligence and wisdom. On a personal level, the sensation of this power growing inside one is a wonderful and stimulating experience. Through it, one acquires self-respect in its best possible meaning. Inner balance and tranquility follow the development of inner strength.

Very often, even a short period of consciously exercising the will and developing inner strength can change an entire life, eventually leading to spiritual rebirth. The path of inner strength is always the right path, but it is not always the one we choose. The Chinese philosopher Chuang-tzu describes a dialogue in which a disciple says to his teacher, "Teacher, we are all men. Why are some men great and some men small?" The teacher answers, "Everyone within himself has two paths, the path of greatness and the path of smallness. If you choose the inner path of greatness, you yourself *might* become a great man, but you will *never* become a great man if you choose the inner path of smallness."

The development of willpower and inner strength leads also to conquering the fears which consciously or unconsciously are an integral part of our psychological makeup, especially as we grow older. Often our lives are ruled by fear—the fear of poverty, ill health, aging, loss of life. The basic fears that we mentioned earlier as connected with aging and the techniques to overcome them will be discussed in more detail in chapter 13 on meditation. The fully evolved person rises above fear, including the fear of death, which gradually can be overcome as the spiritual person is born out of the physical person. The life purified of fear is a new life, much happier, more serene and wholesome, than one at the mercy of fear. Fear can be overcome only by inner strength. Inner strength can be developed only by willpower.

Self-Hypnosis

Sometimes there are particularly difficult habits or attitudes of mind that seem to elude all our conscious attempts to change or influence them: Smoking, overeating, and excessive drinking are among the examples that come readily to mind. In such cases, self-hypnosis can help one to gain control over these compulsive habits. Most of us are probably familiar with the success of hypnosis as practiced by physicians to help people stop smoking or cut down on eating and drinking. With the knowledge of a few techniques, it may be possible for you to perform this service for yourself.

Although hypnosis has been known to mankind for many centuries, it has only recently emerged in the Western world as an accepted tool of medicine. A precise definition of hypnosis still eludes scientific description. Hypnotic trance in its early stages is hardly discernible by the subject. I agree with the school of thought that says hypnosis occurs when there is an accentuated state of suggestibility in the subject. The subject is willing somehow to divert his conscious mind in order that the unconscious may be contacted and activated by the power of suggestion. The predetermined suggestion then gains an influence over the conscious attitude.

Mild forms of self-hypnosis are more familiar than we may think. When an athlete programs himself to be "up" for the performance or game, he is engaging in a highly effective form of self-hypnosis. Actors experience a similar victory over stage fright or loss of memory when they "coach" themselves to perform without distraction. I do not mean to confuse self-hypnosis with concentration; sometimes our concentration on a goal can be enhanced by ritually programming ourselves that we will attain a goal, even if by unorthodox mental approaches. Rituals for "psyching up" the subjects are as old as mankind, as we see in the example of primitive hunters making elaborate ritual preparations before going out for food. We may guess that one purpose of these rituals was to program the psyche so that potential distractions would have no effect.

The susceptibility of the conscious mind to this power of suggestion opens a variety of possibilities for speeding up of healing processes and rejuvenation of cells. It has been demonstrated on many occasions that some diseases that are apparently incurable by orthodox methods will succumb to hypnotic suggestion. Skin diseases are an example.

For many years I have taught self-hypnosis as a means of breaking unwholesome habits and of achieving greater health. Very often my students report that they literally feel younger and healthier even after the first session. One woman told me that her hair started to regain its natural color while brown age spots on her face and hands started to get lighter and disappear after engaging in self-hypnosis. The physiological manifestation of the effects of self-hypnosis is rather unusual in my experience—most people experience a general sense of well-being—yet it is enough to suggest the power inherent in each of us to change our state of health for the better. One of the ancient yogic traditions of rejuvenation gives a very prominent position to self-hypnosis as a means of delaying the aging process. The exercises given below are modified versions of exercises from this tradition.

Prior to engaging in the techniques of self-hypnosis, a number of protective measures should be taken.

First, a person should program his mind regarding the time he intends to spend in the experiment. He should sternly establish in his conscious mind that after a half hour, at a definite clock time, he will be fully awake without any traces of hypnotic trance.

Second, he should make a stern verbal commitment to himself that if any outside interference occurs during his experiment, such as the ringing of the phone or doorbell or the entrance of another person into his room, he will immediately come out of the trance.

Third, another strong verbal statement should program the practicer to discard any suggestion by anyone else who may be present during this experiment. The only voice he should listen to is his own.

Some people are highly vulnerable to suggestion from another person; others resist. The latter may trust his own mind to safeguard any weaknesses and at the same time to influence his behavior in a positive way. Regular practice of the following exercises should bring results in four to six weeks of training, even for the most stubbornly resistant subject. For some, results will occur right away. My recommendation is to try the following exercises if they hold some promise for coping with any difficulties you may be experiencing as a result of weak will. Perhaps autosuggestion will work for you. Be sure to read each exercise through before beginning.

Exercises for Inducing a Mild Hypnotic Trance

1. Lying on your back on the bed or floor, perfectly relaxed and comfortable, with rhythmical and peaceful breath established, concentrate on the sensation of extreme heaviness in the left arm. Convince yourself that your left arm has become so heavy that you are unable to lift it at all. It doesn't matter how hard you try, you simply can't do it. When you feel that you have genuinely achieved that state of heaviness, develop the same sensation in the other arm, the legs, the trunk, the entire body. Try to reach the state wherein you feel that you can't move any limb or raise your body from the supine position. Your mind will be still active and alert; you can hear everything. You are not sleeping, yet you are unable to lift your body off the bed. If you achieve this state, you have induced a hypnotic trance. The fact that you are somewhat awake does not mean that you are not in a trance. Suggestions can then be made (see list below).

2. Another technique is to sit in a cross-legged position on the floor or in a comfortable armchair. Interlace your fingers, close your eyes, establish a rhythmical and peaceful breath. Suggest to yourself that you are unable to separate your fingers— that the more you try to do it, the more tightly knit they become. When you find yourself unable to separate your fingers, it is an indication that you are in a light trance. You can relax completely at that stage and start to work on your psyche with whatever suggestion you want to make.
3. Another method is to imagine that the hands or forehead become cold. As soon as you feel the sensations, you may begin your suggestions.

Beneficial Suggestions That Can Be Made During a Mild Hypnotic Trance

1. If you wish to stop smoking, suggest to yourself that the next time you light a cigarette it won't satisfy you at all; instead of the familiar smell of tobacco, the lit cigarette will emit the most disagreeable smell of burned feathers (or something abhorrent to you) and that you will be unable to take a single puff.
2. If you are having problems with drinking, you can suggest to yourself that in every alcoholic beverage you smell, the very strong odor of turpentine comes through and that you simply won't be able to swallow a drink, even if you try very hard.
3. If eating is a problem, suggest to yourself that as soon as healthy hunger is satisfied you will feel so full that you cannot eat another bite. Reprogram yourself to stop short of overeating.

Beyond these curative effects of controlling unwholesome indulgence, much can be done to delay the aging process. The following are some specific suggestions that can be made while in this state:

1. Direct a command to your sense of personal time to change to a slower pace so that you can experience more relaxation, inner peace, and physical well-being.
2. Command yourself to start thinking young. Henceforth, you will move with greater eagerness to embrace life experience. Your body will reflect this youthful enthusiasm by moving more energetically and gracefully and without fear of brittleness.
3. Command yourself to think positively about your progress through life. The formula "Every day in every way I am getting better and better" should be proclaimed.
4. If you have a specific ailment, concentrate on that and command your diseased part to become whole and well again.

13

Meditation

Just as exercises and breath controls are necessary to the body's health, meditation should be practiced for the health and growth of the psyche. In previous chapters I have shown how keen, alert mental faculties and a well-cared-for body are important to maintaining the balance that we call health. A third component, without which the other two cannot reach their full potential, is spiritual well-being.

Directly and indirectly, meditation plays an important role in delaying aging, and it is an integral part of the three yogas. For centuries, thoughtful people have known that good health and long life depend greatly on spiritual well-being. Yet as we honestly assess our conditions, most of us will find areas of spiritual sterility and stagnation that undermine our attempts at creative life. An important part of the program for rejuvenation includes spiritual renewal through meditation.

All the exercises given in chapter 12 on mental training may be seen as prerequisites to meditation. In meditation, one needs two equally important skills: the ability to think constructively and the ability not to think when thinking becomes a hindrance to some higher aim. Patanjali, with an exactness typical of his genius, defines meditation as "the prolonged holding of the perceiving consciousness to a certain region of attention." He suggests that prolonged concentration on any object or idea will reveal to us the true nature of the object or give us a complete understanding of the idea. When all personal limitations of the perceiving consciousness stand aside, the higher, impersonal mind takes over. The meditator, by transcending his intellect, unites his mind with the universal intelligence and thus enters the highest state of consciousness. This phenomenon is sometimes described as the "flash of genius" that occurs on rare occasions to some human beings; it is the force behind everything created by man on the highest possible level, whether a scientific discovery, a beautiful work of art, or a philosophical revelation.

Meditation is the means by which we can perform the greatest service to our general health; through meditation we get to know ourselves better. We explore our own essential makeup and discover that we are more than a body, even more than a body and a mind.

We cannot become fully rejuvenated unless we cultivate that mysterious part of us that is called "soul" or "psyche" in some philosophical traditions and "the self" in others. These words are not synonymous, and to introduce the word *spirit* may confuse the issue even more, since some philosophies, including yoga, make a distinction between soul and spirit. The soul generally refers to the more personal manifestation of one's essential being, and the spirit to an impersonal spark of divinity within us.

My own belief is that the soul encompasses our mental and moral life, the finest of our aspirations and achievements. The soul's health is regulated by a sense of right and wrong in action and thought—a conscience, if you like. The body lives in the present; the soul lives in the past and in the future. By our actions and thoughts we can impair the body's health and wound the soul; conversely, by appropriate action and thought, we can heal wounds of the soul and body. Attention to the well-being of body, mind, and soul is called "holistic health."

The spirit is the divine spark that exists in each of us, unperturbed by our vacillations. Yet the spirit may remain undiscovered by consciousness until we engage in some form of meditation (either spontaneous or planned). Through meditation we can discover our own immortal essence, or at-oneness with God, the main goal of transcendental meditation.

To simplify matters I am using the terms "spiritual" and "psychic" to refer to that complex association of experiences within the individual that constitute an inner life, through which one becomes aware of one's own soul and of the inner, divine spirit. Mental and physical health depend greatly on our ability to administer to the needs of the soul and to receive the nourishment of the spirit.

Meditation can be defined both as an intense act of reflection and pondering (an intellectual activity) or as a complete absence of thoughts (a cessation of all intellectual activities). These two opposing definitions actually refer to two different types of meditation: intellectual and transcendental. Intellectual meditation is a form of organized thinking that involves the contemplation of subjects and ideas and which leads ultimately to better self-realization as well as greater clarity of thought. Transcendental meditation, on the other hand, is an attempt to go beyond the intellect and reach another plane of consciousness.

Intellectual meditation has prevailed in the West as the main form of creative thinking. Although transcendental meditation has had its own stream in our religious history in the form of Christian illumination, its practice has been mainly confined to mystics. Whenever we have experienced flashes of intuition we have come close to transcendental experience, but our understanding of intuition is severely limited, since we tend to trust only rational thought. Nevertheless, the extent of the Westerner's current interest in Eastern thought and transcendental meditation reflects an apparent readiness to explore altered states of consciousness and to embrace the Eastern concept of the higher mind with some serious intent to develop it.

So far in our culture it is the young who have shown a rapid growth of interest in meditation. I would like to suggest that middle-aged and older people need more than anyone else to become champions of the philosophic mind, whether on an intellectual or transcendental plane.

In preparing for meditation, our first task is to become aware of the enormous influence of spiritual health over general health. I have witnessed several impressive examples of the way psychic shock or stress can "age" a person, causing wrinkles where none appeared before, gray hair in the place of the natural color, and a general shrunken appearance in the body. The Russian poet F. Tutcheff reportedly aged several years in twenty-four hours when his wife died.

For most of us who experience stress, the changes are not so dramatic, yet stress takes a gradual toll on our youthfulness, especially if we lack the ability to take it in stride or to "bounce back" from sudden shocks. This ability does not come easily because our culture does not teach us much about handling stress.

The gains that have been made in science and technology in the West have paradoxically produced a situation in which we often find ourselves serving technology instead of the other way around. Human values need to be reasserted in the West so that science and technology

become our servants instead of our masters. No enlightened scientist wishes to mechanize human beings, yet
when we observe the gridlike layout of our cities with
their high-rise buildings which all look so much alike,
and when we get the message time and time again that
it is not our individuality that matters but rather our
ability to conform our lives to serve the needs of industry,
we can only conclude that we live in a world that values
products more than it values people. We are constantly
subjected to rapid changes in our environment, a hurried
pace of existence, relentless pressure in work and social
life. The main antidote we are offered against the anxieties produced by these factors is drugs, and one of the
main problems for a large portion of our population is
the growing dependency on drugs. Unfortunately, we
tend to focus our attention on the problem of drug abuse
among the young while ignoring the culturally condoned
form of addiction to painkillers and antidepressants that
disables adults of all ages.

To grow older, for many people, is to feel more and
more helpless, vulnerable to misfortunes of all kinds, subject to miscellaneous elusive aches and pains as well as
specific diseases, often unable to sleep or to sleep well,
likely to carry anxiety over from one situation to another,
and to suffer frequent bouts of depression. One can gain
temporary relief from these maladies by taking drugs
of one kind or another, but when the effect of the drug
wears off, the anxiety or pain is likely to return. And,
of course, many drugs have detrimental side effects. Most
of all, however, being under the influence of drugs prevents us from being truly ourselves. Instead of achieving
greater self-awareness and spiritual independence as we
mature, we may become more dependent and even lose
touch with sources of inner strength.

Many people are now in the process of rejecting the

self-image of the "consumer of products," including drugs—an image that has been so carefully inculcated by modern advertising. Yoga, which is deeply humanistic in philosophy, can play a tremendously important role in this readjusting of the psyche. Through yoga we can reestablish the basic integrity of mind, body, and soul on the individual level. We must keep ourselves alive and well whether or not doing so is good for the tobacco or drug industry, to use only two of many possible examples. This attitude might be called "creative selfishness," and it is the proper antidote to those who appeal to our very patriotism to literally kill ourselves for the sake of modern industry.

Meditation offers a way to loose ourselves from such dependencies by becoming more aware of our natural and innate growth patterns and by helping us to find a personal path toward "the good life"—one that contributes to health, productivity, satisfaction, and serenity. It is a time-tested alternative to drugs—whether they be of the mind-expanding or tranquilizing varieties. Perhaps most importantly, it is the door to spiritual growth and cosmic realization, the highest goal of humankind.

Essentially, we all know what is good for us and what is bad for us. There is an indwelling, intuitive voice of wisdom that every one of us can consult for every decision we make. This voice is suppressed much of the time in order that we may do what others expect of us instead of what we know is right. By habitually ignoring this voice, which I like to refer to as "the little guru within," the voice becomes weaker and weaker until finally we cannot hear it at all. When we dismiss this voice as if it were the buzz of an annoying fly, we jeopardize our health and shorten our life expectancy. If we refuse to listen to it, our bodies punish us with aches and pains, warning signals of more serious danger to come. Finally, we may succumb to serious illness or even death.

In this chapter I present some basic practices in meditation that I believe are highly beneficial in relieving some of the adverse symptoms of aging and in achieving spiritual renewal, all of which contribute to the likelihood of total rebirth as I describe it in this book.

The best time for meditation is early morning or evening. It should be practiced in quiet surroundings with no distractions. Meditation should never be practiced on a full stomach or after imbibing alcohol.

A few minutes should be spent experimenting with breathing until the right rhythm (one that satisfies the meditator at that particular time) is found. Sometimes a gentle breath is most satisfying, as it produces no sound and is not distracting. Different schools of meditation advocate different techniques of breathing during meditation. The Chinese school, for instance, advocates the breath which hugs the upper, inner walls of both nostrils, stimulating the upper cortex of the brain, for intellectual meditation. Deep and rhythmical breathing is a widely recommended breath control for meditation. All schools agree that a thorough study of breath controls should precede meditative practices. Only then can one choose the most satisfactory method for supporting the mind with breath.

The ability to sit cross-legged and motionless for at least half an hour is also very important. If, for some reason, the cross-legged pose is unsatisfactory, a comfortable chair could be used. It should not be so comfortable as to encourage dozing, however.

MEDITATION 1: Sorting of Thoughts and Values

In the process of mental and spiritual development, it is very important to be able to create a scale of values, discarding all that is second- or third-rate or worthless, and assimilating the essence of our experiences. This ability to sort, or sift, should be brought to the most mundane of our experiences when we can't avoid the mundane altogether. For instance, it is not always possible to choose the conversations we will hear, but it is possible to tune out meaningless chatter and to really listen only to what we want to assimilate. It is possible to avoid many commitments that we know beforehand will lead us nowhere or, when we do keep commitments, to search for meaning and purpose in them.

One experience that remains vivid to me occurred one morning when my Chinese master brought an artichoke into the meditation room. We had been waiting for him, as always, since early in the morning. When he entered, he sat down in his place facing us, produced the artichoke, contemplated it for a few seconds, and then, slowly, deliberately, started to remove the leaves one by one, placing them in a neat pile. When he reached the heart of the artichoke, he contemplated it again for a long moment, then he got up and walked away. We did not understand his "message." The next day he did exactly the same thing. Awkward and ashamed, again we couldn't perceive the meaning of the action. On the third day he explained to us that in the process of living we accumulate layers of personality which very often obscure our real selves. The real self is the heart of an artichoke, but to get to it you must learn how to remove the layers of surface.

The ability to know what is you essentially and what is not you is the theme of this meditation. We often hear the expression "That is not you." "It can't be you." "Your real self is incapable of acting in this or that particular way." These are indications from outside us that we behave in ways that are strange or inappropriate to the "self" that are sometimes recognized by our intimates even when we are not aware of the subtle changes.

Sorting is a fundamental practice of intellectual meditation. Begin by finding your most satisfying meditative
pose. Close your eyes and imagine that you hold in your
hand an artichoke. Begin to remove the leaves, trying
to connect each leaf with some aspect of yourself or some
value that you hold. Continue until you have taken away
all the outer manifestations of your personality, including
shallow values, and have gotten down to the core or heart
of yourself. Reaching this "center" will give you a sense
of freedom and immortality, of liberation from the mundane in yourself and in the world.

MEDITATION 2: Purification of Thoughts and Emotions
   One cannot become fully rejuvenated without re-
creating one's moral health through purification of actions, thoughts, and emotions. Of course, it is generally
recommended that in our actions we refrain from behavior that is either self-destructive or harmful to others.
Meditation on purification of thoughts and emotions has
a beneficial effect on actions, too.
   Philosophies the world over designate certain human
tendencies that must constantly be purged if we are to
achieve rebirth. To be filled with negative emotions like
envy, jealousy, anger, lust, and pride (we have referred
to the other two of the seven deadly sins—sloth and glut-
tony—in chapter 7) is to live in a turmoil that will not
permit liberation of the spirit. At best, these are all prisons
of pettiness; we must be liberated from them if we are
to experience the larger and more satisfying life rewards.
   Purification involves not only reeducating negative
tendencies from one's present habits of mind and heart
but also a reasonable atonement for past shortcomings
and the "letting go" of undue and ineffective remorse
where no retribution is possible. Positive remorse, like
true grief, is a form of meaningful suffering and has a

beneficial effect on the spirit; negative or useless remorse is debilitating.

There are many themes for meditation in this category. The following are suggested to get you started—others will suggest themselves as you follow this path.

Find a satisfactory meditative pose and close your eyes. Breathe deeply and rhythmically. Concentrate on exploring your psyche for evidence of any tendencies toward anger or hatred. Try to identify clearly the object of this emotion, the issues involved, and the causes. After clarifying the situation as best you can, work on convincing yourself that hatred is a negative and self-destructive quality and that you must liberate yourself from it for your own sake, if not that of others. Teach yourself that before you can fully and freely like or love another, you must learn how not to dislike or hate. Focus on the latter. Say to yourself, "I will now cease giving energy to this wasteful negative emotion." Once you are able to stop the flow of energy in a negative direction, you can use that energy in a more positive way. Consider how you might do that as a final step in this meditation. *How can I redirect this energy?* Perhaps you will want simply to relax from the strain of active dislike.

One can proceed systematically through a list of negative thoughts and emotions, exploring them, ceasing to contribute energy to them, relaxing, and redirecting energy.

This same series of meditations can be continued to explore the opposite of the negative emotion. If hatred is debilitating, love is energizing. It is the force that binds or joins all things in harmonious relationship. It is the force that some philosophies identify with God ("God is love").

One can easily see how such a simple beginning with attention to the negative aspects of one's character can lead one ultimately to the supreme purification of the soul: the identification of one's own spirit with divinity, from which experience one does not easily return to base emotions or thoughts.

One should also spend some meditative time exploring feelings of guilt and remorse. We are often involuntarily subjected to these feelings. One way to gain control of them is to invite them voluntarily into a meditation, to identify their sources when possible, to ask whether we have done all we can to atone for the incidents which caused them, to resolve to take any steps left open for atonement, and then to banish the feelings resolutely. Again, the key is to stop contributing vital energy to a worthless cause.

MEDITATION 3: Handling Stress

In the introduction I mentioned the stress of modern life as a source of anxiety from which many people suffer, sometimes mildly, sometimes severely. Stress is certainly one of the main factors in premature aging. I have already indicated in a general way that meditation can relieve stress. Regular meditation on any of the subjects given in this chapter will alleviate many anxieties. The key to coping with stress is not to avoid anxiety, which is a natural reaction to a threatening situation, but rather to relax and resume normal functioning after a threat has passed. Many people continue to manifest the symptoms of anxiety (accelerated heartbeat, tensed muscles) long after the cause is removed, and so build from one threatening situation to another an accumulation of fatigue and tension from the unrelieved burden.

One meditation for relieving stress is similar to those for purifying oneself of negative thoughts and emotions. Seat yourself comfortably, close your eyes, breathe deeply and rhythmically. The deep breathing will have an immediate beneficial effect, since anxiety tends to result in shallow, quick breathing. Deliberately slowing the breath will help you to gain control over other bodily responses. Practice the breathing for relaxation exercises described in chapter 5 on breathing. Once you have attained a relaxed meditative posture, try to identify the source of your anxiety. Is it a real threat to your essential well-being? Then reflect on ways to combat the threat. Is it an imaginary threat—a worry over something that might happen? Many things that we worry over never materialize, and we waste precious energy in dreaded anticipation. Many people, especially older people, are a constant prey to "catastrophic expectation"—they expect the worst when the odds are at least half in favor of a more promising outcome. Try honestly to assess the dreaded situation and come to terms with it. Then let it go. Give yourself a conscious directive to "flow" with whatever happens. You can do no more, and by consciously adapting yourself to a situation, you will stand a much greater chance of emerging intact—perhaps even strengthened by it.

MEDITATION 4: Transforming Fears

In chapter 2 on the mental symptoms of aging I mentioned certain fears that plague people as they grow older. Fear has a powerfully adverse effect on the psyche and the body that can be relieved through meditation. Here are subjects for meditation based on each of these major fears. The pose and attitude should be the same as recommended at the beginning of the chapter.

Fear of Losing Possessions

One of the delightful stories I heard in China that has a message worthy of meditation tells of a traveler who saw a ruined house—apparently, it had just burned down. Strangely, an old man gleefully played a flute and danced around the house. Amazed, the traveler asked the man why he seemed so happy. The old man replied, "Once I possessed no property and I was extremely happy. Through circumstances, I again have no property. I see no reason why I shouldn't be happy." The realization that true happiness is a state of mind which has little connection to material possessions liberates one from the fear of losing possessions.

Fear of Losing Health

The most important aspect of meditation on the physical body is that it brings accentuated awareness of our physical nature; that leads to mastery over bodily functions and thus to healthier living, meanwhile relieving one of fear of falling sick. Meditation on health allows one to acquire deep in his psyche the belief that he is responsible for his own physical well-being and that he is capable of maintaining his body in the right balance. One consequently gains a certain amount of mastery over his body which can even exclude the possibility of falling ill. Of course, no one, not even a yogi, is immune from illness. However, if one has the right attitude, even if some ailment does befall (in the case of the yogi, illness is believed to be due most often to karmic influences), one can react to it with inner strength and dignity.

Fear of Aging

The fear of aging, with all its likely adverse manifestations, is one of the themes of this book. One of the most important tasks to be met by the aging person is the challenge of time's effects on the body, mind, and spirit.

Meditation should include a contemplation of various aspects of aging as they affect you and the gradual conquering of these effects deep in your psyche by creative thought and imagery, especially as it relates to a more youthful, vital, dynamic person within yourself. Locate the areas of physical deterioration as they manifest themselves in your own body, and transform these effects first through imagizing the converse tendencies. "As a person thinks, so is he" can be a useful guideline for these meditations, which should also include contemplation of the mental and spiritual signs of aging in yourself and work on reversing them.

Through meditation, aging can be delayed. It can be looked upon, not as a humiliating process of physical and mental deterioration, but as a gradual unfolding of the spiritual man or woman out of the physical one.

Fear of Loneliness

"When all other doors are closed to you, the door to inner space remains open." This is my philosophy about loneliness. We live in a culture that is basically extraverted, so much so that we find it difficult to admit that we may be our own best company. Friendship is a generous gift of the gods, and I don't mean to deny even in the minutest sense its value. Yet I do think it important to profess that the company of one's own private self is also a gift of the gods and that it offers the unique experience of unification with cosmic consciousness through meditation. When journeying into inner space, one comes closest to God. Inner space is the sphere that links us to the matrix and goal of our lives. Meditation on this inward path can transform the yearning of loneliness into the fulfillment of inner adventure.

Fear of Death

The prevalent attitude toward death in our culture is one of fear and denial. It has always seemed strange to me that death should be a taboo subject when the experience offers two rather attractive alternatives: It could be either a much-needed repose or the greatest of adventures. Both prospects are deeply satisfying to the psyche, provided one has lived out his potential for creative and noble behavior in this life. Only where one remains attached to this embodiment through guilt over mismanaged personal relationships or unrealized potential does one view death as the end of everything. Truly, it is the end of one's opportunities to atone for misdeeds or to have adventures in this life; therefore, the prospect of death is to be taken seriously, even if you believe in reincarnation—perhaps especially if you do.

Personally, I am not unduly dismayed by the prospect of a long repose, but I believe that is not the likeliest prospect of death. There is too much evidence from prophets, poets, and scientists that death is the portal to a much vaster experience.

The entire Eastern metaphysical tradition teaches that a man experiences two great events during his present life: his coming into the world and his going out from it. In this tradition, and in the tradition of many religions of the world, physical expiration is the beginning of new life, on an entirely different plane unknown to us in our living state. From the philosophical point of view, the second part of man's life is, in a way, a continuous preparation for his death. It has nothing to do with the morbid fascination for death, but it is awareness of the liberation of one's better part into the new world.

The subject for meditation along these lines is the metaphor given by nature in the caterpillar-cocoon-butterfly triad. We can see our earthly existence as comparable to that of the caterpillar, who is ignorant of his real nature. The cocoon represents the death state, which is really not a death but a preparation for life on a different plane. The mysterious transformation of the ugly worm into the beautiful butterfly is the most vivid example of the difference between our lower and higher selves. Leaving behind its primitive physical form, the butterfly, a symbol for the psyche or soul, spreads its wings into the beautiful sun-penetrated ether. Regular meditation of this sort will liberate one's mind from the fear of death, bringing the meditator closer and closer to the realization of his or her true self, which is immortal and divine in its essence.

14

Eighty-four Steps to Rebirth[1]

At the beginning of the book I told the story of a master who was able to grow a new body. During almost fifty years of my pursuit of esoteric knowledge, I came across only three cases in which yogis attempted the growing of a new body. The one I described was a success. The other two attempts ended in death. To grow a new body first requires the arduous and extremely dangerous task of reducing the old body almost to skin and bones and then regrowing it, atom by atom, through breath controls as well as special diets, exercises, and meditations. My intention in this chapter is not to elaborate on this mysterious method, which is best left to Eastern ascetics of long tradition and training, but to present a method of rejuvenation that can be embarked upon with a reasonable expectation of success by the Western student.

In the Eastern tradition, seekers after enlightenment are divided into four categories, according to their degree of dedication, their character, their willingness to learn and to sacrifice. These categories of people are (1) feeble, (2) average, (3) superior, and (4) supreme. Superior seek-

1. This is a very important chapter as it summarizes a definitive plan for counteracting the aging process. Dedicated students following this plan could experience rebirth on spiritual, mental, and physical levels.

ers are rare, supreme ones even rarer. However, as I asserted earlier, with concentrated desire, anything is possible. So even if we begin in the feeble or average stage, we may achieve remarkable results.

It is possible at any point in life to turn back the biological clock—to improve health and the general condition of the body to such a dramatic degree that one feels reborn. The most visible progress can be seen in cases of elderly people who literally can win for themselves a second lease on life, with many more years of creative work and pleasure. No matter how worn-out or rundown you may feel at present, you can wake up one morning with the sensations of having restored your youthful vitality, grace, and attractiveness, as well as an adventurous mind and spirit. That is what I mean by rebirth.

Throughout this book I have presented many ways of cultivating body, mind, and soul for the purpose of achieving a longer and healthier life. Many of these techniques can be learned readily by the student. Presumably you will have already begun to follow suggestions in the previous chapters for obtaining the benefits of wholesome diet, adequate sleep, contact with nature, assimilation of energy through breath control, shaping the body, and toning the skin. You should also have begun mental training exercises and meditations. For the truly ambitious student, this chapter will present a rigorous program that, if followed closely, can result in total renewal, both physically and spiritually. I believe that this renewal or rebirth can be achieved in eighty-four steps (outlined below) by anyone who is dedicated and who follows the guidance as well of "the guru within" who will help you to design cycles of exercises that are best suited to your needs.

I learned much of this method for rejuvenation in an island ashram of my Taoist master in China. It is a carefully blended mixture of techniques from three yogas.

The eighty-four steps include seven purifying processes for the body, seven breath controls, seven body-sculpting gestures, seven techniques designed to stimulate the inner life of the body, seven meditative practices, and forty-nine bodily postures.[2]

Many techniques given in this chapter are much more challenging than anything that has been done by the student so far. Nevertheless, many dedicated people will be able to master most (perhaps all) of these techniques. Most of them are greater challenges to the willpower than to the body. Some of the *asanas,* or bodily positions, will demand rigorous adherence to a daily routine that encourages gradual success. Among my students there are men and women who have mastered every bodily pose as late as in their sixties. Mastery of a pose is defined as that point when the pose is performed without difficulty or strain, and the flow of breath is undisturbed during its execution. The battle is long and strenuous. The least time required to achieve impressive results is nine months of daily physical training, meditation, breath controls, and disciplines of diet and sleep.

Any Westerner embarking on such a program as I recommend here has two major problems to overcome: One is the lack of a tradition which might offer psychological support and even an appropriate setting (such as an ashram) for the venture; another is a normal daily routine which does not permit time or leisure to carry out such a program. Nevertheless, I have given much thought to my experiences with students in various parts of the world

2. In the metaphysical tradition, the number seven is the most important number. There are seven chakras in the body, seven various "bodies" of a person, eighty-four traditional *asanas* (a multiple of seven), forty-nine points used in Chinese breath controls related to physical, mental, and spiritual well-being (again, a multiple of seven). There are seven rays in the spectrum, seven notes in a musical scale. Many breathing rhythms have a ratio of seven. In Sufi traditions, there are many sayings related to the "seventh heaven."

where I have taught and lectured. I am convinced that satisfying results can be achieved by a person who is prepared to spend one hour or so in daily practice—half an hour in the morning and another half hour in the evening; of course, the more time spent, the better.

A suggested daily and weekly regime is as follows: The morning routine (before taking any food or liquid) should include *each day* the seven purifying processes (they can become a normal part of your bathroom procedure), with the *mudra* called *uddiyan* performed to aid elimination. Daily morning practices should also include the seven body-sculpting gestures which require only about five minutes and which, if practiced with absolute regularity each day at the same time, will tone and strengthen every major group of body muscles. Of the seven breath controls, three should be practiced daily and rotated with the others. Of the seven meditations, one should be practiced each morning and rotated with the others.

The rest of the program should be carried out in the evening when you are free of duties. The evening routine should begin with the limbering-up movements described in chapter 8 on shaping the body. These should be followed by stretching and twisting exercises and by at least three inverted positions: shoulder stand, pose of longevity, and headstand (if possible). If time permits, all seven inverted postures should be practiced on a daily basis.

After this regular daily schedule, one should determine what other exercises should be added to serve personal needs. Specific weaknesses, such as stiffness in some joints of the body, should be countered with exercises designed to make that area more supple. Add as many exercises as time and dedication permit until you are satisfied that your daily routine will bring you gradually to the goal of total renewal. Each experience of improvement is a great incentive to continue your progress, and every mastered technique is one step closer to the experience of rebirth.

Seven Purifying Processes

These should be done at the beginning of each day as follows:

1. Elimination, which is aided by regular practice of abdominal contraction known as *uddiyan,* then moving *uddiyan,* then *nauli* (see pp. 85–87 for reference to descriptions of these *mudras)* to promote vigorous massage of the entire digestive area. These techniques not only lead to elimination of impurities on a regular basis, but they encourage a complete emptying of the digestive tract as the powerful flapping of the abdominal muscles forces impurities down the colon and out.
2. A careful cleaning of the anus, using toilet paper, followed by a water cleansing of the anal area. One theory concerning cancer of the rectum is that it could be traced to inadequate cleansing of the anus. In women, infections are sometimes spread from the anal area to the sexual or urinary channels if the anus is not kept meticulously clean.
3. Washing the entire body either by bath, shower, or sponging.
4. Cleaning the teeth.
5. Removing impurities from the tongue. Hygiene of the mouth includes gently removing impurities that have accumulated overnight on the tongue by a spoon, the blunt end of a nail file, or any similar instrument. If impurities are not removed

from the tongue in the morning, they are reab-
sorbed into the system with the first drink or food.
6. Washing the nostrils. Regular cleaning of the nostrils makes the process of breathing easier and
more pleasant; it checks the accumulation of impurities in the nasal passages, prevents sinus con-
gestion and infection as well as colds in the head
and throat.

Mix one-quarter teaspoon of salt with warm
water in a tumbler. Closing one nostril, inhale the
water through the other nostril until it starts to
flow out from the mouth. The process is repeated
several times for both nostrils.
7. Washing the eyes. This is the most unorthodox
of all the cleansing processes recommended, but
if done with discretion, it is rewarding. The technique consists of staring without blinking at a single point on the wall (a small black dot can be
painted there). Then the eyes are opened as wide
as possible, closed tightly, then blinked several
times. This activates tear glands. The eyes are thus
washed with one's own tears.
Note: As an additional discipline benefiting the
facial skin, I would suggest splashing the face with
cold water mixed with the juice of one-quarter
lemon.

Seven *Mudras* and *Bandhas*

The seven *mudras,* some of them identified as *bandhas*
by masters of yoga, play an important part in achieving
rebirth and then maintaining radiant health. They include those "inverted gymnastics," or exercises for inner
organs, which tone up the digestive and eliminative powers of the body as well as stimulate the nervous centers

and endocrine glands. They reveal the most profound knowledge regarding the functioning and physical well-being of the human body. Nothing as yet in the Western tradition even comes close to the ingenuity of these techniques. In the Tibetan tradition they are said to be designed not by men but by higher entities who passed them to men as a gift from heaven. See Glossary for reference to descriptions of each of the following:

1. *Uddiyan bandha*
2. *Jalandhara bandha*
3. *Mula bandha*
4. *Maha mudra*
5. *Yoga mudra*
6. *Mahavedha mudra*
7. *Prana-apana mudra*

Seven Body-Sculpting Movements

In an urban society, our daily activities are not sufficient to tone up many groups of muscles in our bodies. That is why, in attaining ultimate rebirth, body isometrics, backed by the creative power of the mind, play such an important part. Of the body-sculpting movements related to twelve regions of the body described earlier in chapter 8 on shaping the body, seven are considered the most important. These also should be practiced at the same time every day.

Exercise 1 (arms and shoulders)
Exercise 3 (sides and back)
Exercise 4 (chest and abdomen)
Exercise 7 (back, shoulders, and chest)
Exercise 8 (back chest, and buttocks)
Exercise 11 (tiptoes)
Exercise 12 (all muscles)

Seven *Pranayamas*

Of the *pranayamas* described in chapter 5 on breathing exercises, seven are the most important to achieve rebirth and to maintain health. They are as follows; three of them should be practiced on a daily basis, while the other four should be done in rotation:

1. Snake Breath (for rejuvenating facial skin). Daily.
2. Blacksmith Bellows (a blood purifier). Daily.
3. Cooling Breath (for lowering the temperature of the body and leading to longevity). Daily.
4. Energy Breath using alternate nostrils (for toning the sympathetic nervous system).
5. *Anahata Pranayama* (breath and meditation upon the cardiac plexus for slowing down the biological clock).
6. Bee, producing the mantra of health (for toning up vital organs through vibration).
7. Gentle Breath (for slowing down the biological clock and conveying the sensation of lightness).

Forty-Nine *Asanas*

Relaxed Positions

Seemingly undemanding, the seven relaxed positions in fact are very difficult to perfect and should be worked at assiduously.

EXERCISE 1: *Savasana* (Complete Relaxation)
    Traditionally, this position precedes other training. In it the student is not only relaxing and recharging his body with energy, but he is readjusting his psyche by attuning himself to appropriate vibrations.

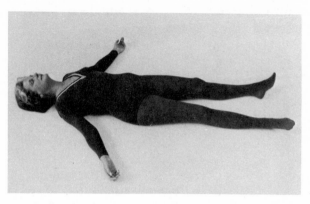

Art of complete relaxation lying on the back (*Savasana*)

This exercise is performed while lying on the back, preferably on a mat or on a firm bed, with the feet slightly apart and arms alongside the body, palms up. *Savasana* consists of four stages:

1. Relax the muscles gradually, from the tip of the toes upward to feet and ankles, calves, knees, thighs, hips, abdomen, small of the back, chest, shoulders, arms, hands; finally, the facial muscles are completely relaxed (you may be astonished at the amount of tension there) by sagging the lower jaw, relaxing the forehead, and loosening facial muscles. The tongue can be relaxed, as well as the eyeballs in their sockets—even the muscles of the skull.

   Upon achieving complete relaxation of the muscles of the body, the mind's eye is turned inward in search of possible tension. Additional effort and concentration should be exercised to produce complete relaxation of the entire nervous system.

2. Concentrate on emptying the *nadis,* or nervous-psychic channels, of the body to prepare them

for being recharged by pranic force through deep and rhythmical breathing.

3. Recharge the body through deep and rhythmical breathing. Visualize *prana* drawn into your system with incoming breath and directed through thousands of *nadis* to every living cell of the body with outgoing breath. It is taught that if complete relaxation is achieved, only twelve slow and deep breaths are sufficient to create the sensation of being recharged.

4. The final part of *savasana* is described in the metaphysical teachings as a "small exit" from the physical body, an escape into a different world, unrelated and detached from the present environment. Imagine yourself in a beautiful garden thousands of miles away, surrounded by great beauty, happy, relaxed, and secure.

I learned about escaping into a beautiful garden during my training in Taoist yoga in China. One of the ashrams where I stayed was ancient, partly dilapidated, but surrounded by the most lovely garden full of rare trees, flowering bushes, ponds, and meditative shrines. It was a tradition that a new student entering the ashram should bring a rare tree or long-lived shrub to be planted on the day of his arrival to commemorate the beginning of his training. It is easy to see that over a period of hundreds of years some of these gardens consisted of the most beautiful and rare plants imaginable.

As a part of the discipline and sometimes as "meditation in action," every inhabitant of the ashram spent at least two hours daily working in the garden. People with artistic talents and skilled stonemasons landscaped various parts of the gardens or built scenic little bridges or shrines, while others engaged in more mundane work such as sweeping and tidying the garden or cultivating vegetable patches. When a student was to leave the ashram, the teacher would take him for a final round, walking with him hand in hand and saying the traditional farewell incantation: "When you will be far away, lonesome, or longing to relax, close your eyes and come back to this garden. Even if I am dead, I will be waiting for you."

Even without the actual experience described above, the student can use his imagination to create an image of a beautiful garden—a mental retreat or sanctuary which provides complete relaxation for the mind, creating the sensation of complete detachment from all problems.

EXERCISE 2: Yoga *Nidra*

This exercise is also practiced while in the supine position. As in the previous exercise, outer and inner relaxation are achieved first and then rhythmical breath is established. The student learns how to detach himself gradually from the sensation of his physical body, putting his entire awareness into the process of breathing. He learns how to achieve this bit by bit, detaching himself first from the sensation of his left leg, then his right arm, his right leg, left arm, and eventually his entire body. When his consciousness dwells completely in respiration, he is trained to concentrate on three states: (1) lightness, (2) transparency, (3) bodilessness. When each sensation has been experienced, the final state is prolonged for 5–10 minutes. It is beautifully refreshing and recharging on all planes.

EXERCISE 3

Complete relaxation is achieved while lying on the right side in the natural and relaxed position of a sleeping person—body slightly curled, knees slightly bent, right arm stretched above the head with the head resting on it, left arm resting on the hip or behind the back. Breathing is deep and rhythmical, as closely resembling sleeping breath as possible.

EXERCISE 4

This exercise is the reverse of the previous one, but lying this time on the left side.

EXERCISE 5: *Advasana*

Relaxation on the stomach. The head should be turned to the right or left side, arms at the sides of the body, feet slightly apart, toes stretched out. Breathing is deep and rhythmical.

This exercise is a very important sleeping pose, as it teaches the student how to relax completely, conscious or asleep. Incidentally, when sleeping this way, one should have a firm mattress and should not use a pillow.

EXERCISE 6: Pose of a Child

Kneeling, with feet pointed straight behind, resting the hips on the heels, the body is folded in the shape of a fetus, with the arms stretching back alongside the feet. It is astonishing during this pose how many tensions must be eliminated before achieving the perfectly relaxed attitude. The ability to enjoy this position also includes the right weight of the body. An overweight person or a person with a protruding stomach, as well as one with stiff ankles, is not able fully to enjoy this *asana*. Breathing should be natural.

EXERCISE 7: Modified Pose of a Fish

This exercise is done on the back with the legs crossed and heels drawn up close to the body while knees are completely relaxed, dropping sideways. Arms are folded

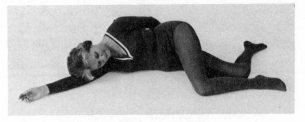

Lying on the side—right and left aspects (*Savasana*)

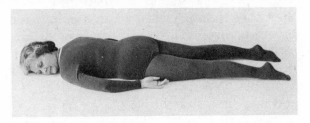

Prone position (*Advasana*)

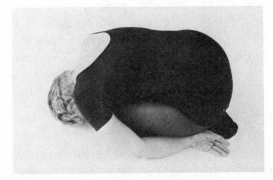

Pose of a Child

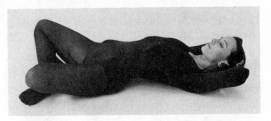

Modified pose of a fish (*Ardha-Matsyasana*)

behind the head, with the left hand under the right shoulder and the right hand under the left shoulder. Apart from being a pleasant position for relaxation, this is a wonderful pose to experience full abdominal breathing spontaneously.

Seated Positions

These positions should be mastered completely, since they play an important part in meditative practices and breath controls. The four cross-legged positions are described earlier in chapter 5 on breathing exercises. Apart from these, seated positions include the following (in all these positions special emphasis is given to keeping back and neck in a straight line):

EXERCISE 5: Thunderbolt Pose *(Vajrasana)*
Sometimes known as the diamond pose, this one consists of sitting with the back and neck in a straight line over the back of the heels. This position is greatly beneficial for knees and insteps, keeping legs from rheumatic disorders, and it is conducive to mental peace and tranquility. It is widely used as a meditative pose in Zen Buddhism, often in preference to the cross-legged poses.

EXERCISE 6: Pose of a Hero *(Virasana)*
In this seated position, one leg is bent backward away from the body while the other foot is placed on the opposite thigh close to the groin as in the lotus position. Back and neck are in a straight line. Eyes are either closed or concentrated on the tip of the nose. Breathing is deep and rhythmical.

This position, according to tradition, was taught to Alexander the Great by yogis in India. It is used for meditative and contemplative practices as well as in mental training where inner strength and willpower are developed.

Thunderbolt Pose (*Vajrasana*)

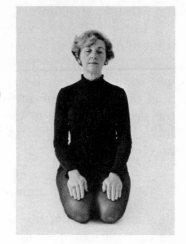

Pose of a Hero (*Virasana*)

Half Lotus Pose (*Ardhapadmasana*)

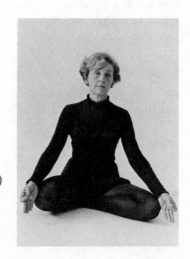

EXERCISE 7: Half Lotus *(Ardhapadmasana)*

In the half lotus position, which, to a certain extent, resembles the pose of the adept, the right or left heel is placed close to the *yoni* place (between anus and genitals) while the other foot is raised as in the lotus position, high up on the opposite thigh, with the heel touching the groin. It is one of the natural cross-legged poses of India, and in the yoga tradition it is used for meditative practices.

Balancing Exercises

Regular practice of the balancing exercises plays an important part in delaying a certain aspect of the aging process. The sense of balance reaches its peak rather early in life (perhaps as early as in the teens) and gradually deteriorates; in older years it is almost completely lost without regular training to keep it. That is why old people are so insecure in their movements, in walking, and generally in controlling their bodies. The practice of balancing seems to reverse this aspect of aging and in many cases to restore completely the sense of balance. Balancing exercises naturally improve the sense of concentration as well. All balancing exercises contribute to inner balance. In physiotherapy, balancing exercises are often used to treat cases of brain damage, including those resulting from alcohol abuse. Most of the exercises are done with the eyes closed. The balancing exercises vary greatly, from those that are simple to learn to difficult and more demanding ones. They all should eventually be mastered.

EXERCISE 1: Pose of a Tree *(Vrikshasana)*

This consists of standing alternatively on one leg (and then the other) with the other foot pressed against the inside of the opposite knee, with the hands in an attitude of prayer in front of the chest. Breath is rhythmical. Eyes are concentrated on the tip of the nose or on a point on the ground some 4 feet away. Starting from only a few seconds, try to increase the balance stance to an indefinite time without much difficulty.

EXERCISE 2: Standing Half Lotus

This one is performed by standing on one foot with the other one in the half lotus attitude, heel close to the groin, knee down, arms above head, palms joined. Other directions are as above.

EXERCISE 3: Dancing Pose *(Natarajasana)*

While standing on one leg, the opposite foot is grasped by the corresponding hand while the other arm is raised up in the air in a gesture of salutation. Breath, eye concentration, and duration are the same as above.

EXERCISE 4: Pose of an Eagle *(Garudasana)*

Considerably more demanding than the previous three exercises. While standing on the right leg, with the knees slightly bent, the left leg is wound over the right leg and under so that the left toes grasp the inside of the right calf. Arms repeat the movement of the legs in the opposite direction, right elbow over left, hands reaching until they clasp. Elbows are brought to knees, eyes concentrated on the tip of the nose, breath deep and rhythmical.

Apart from developing the sense of balance, this position promotes limberness in the joints of the arms and legs. It is favored by celibate yogis because it supposedly sublimates sexual energy.

EXERCISE 5: Balancing on the Toes

This balancing pose requires the ability to balance on the tip of the toes with the arms raised and fingertips touching above the head. It is practiced using both feet

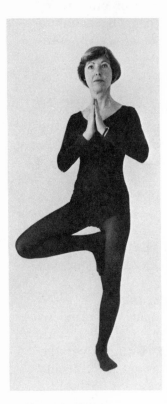

Pose of a Tree

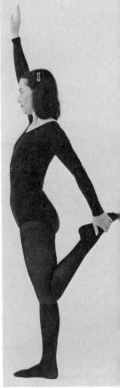

Dancing Pose
(*Natarajasana*)

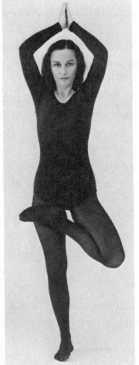

Standing Half Lotus

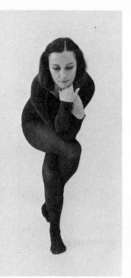

Pose of an Eagle
(*Garudasana*)

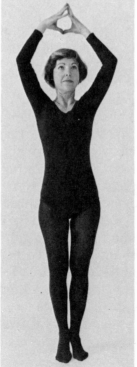

Squatting Pose
(*Padangushtasana*)

Balancing on the Toes

in the beginning for balance, and then on the right and left foot alternatively. The final objective of this exercise is to be able to retain balance on either foot for the duration of 6 heartbeats with the eyes closed. Breathing and eye concentration are the same as above.

EXERCISE 6: Squatting Pose *(Padangushtasana)*

Squatting is done on the tip of the toes. Back and neck are kept in a straight line. Hands rest on the knees and eyes concentrate on the tip of the nose. Breath is deep and rhythmical as in the other positions. Retention of this position is for 12 deep breaths; then return to original position.

A variation is to squat with the heels on the floor, a more demanding position than on the toes. The ability to squat on the right and left foot alternately is even more difficult. Only one squatting position is necessary to this cycle; the others are mentioned as refinements.

EXERCISE 7: Knee-Foot Pose *(Vatayanasana)*

The most demanding of all balancing poses requires that the student balance on one knee and one foot. The other foot is brought against the thigh as in the lotus position. The easiest way to learn this position is to sit down on the floor with the legs outstretched. The right or left leg is bent, and the heel is brought close to the groin as in the lotus position. Then the other leg is bent and foot is put flat on the floor close to the body, using hands in the beginning to help to get into this final position. Upon establishing it, put the hands in an attitude of prayer in front of the chest. Breath is deep and rhythmical. The position is retained on the right and left sides for the duration of 12 heartbeats.

This pose requires extreme limberness of the foot and knee joints while pressure in the region of the groin stim-

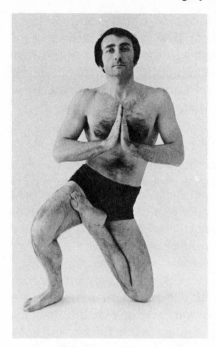

Knee-Foot Pose (*Vatayanasana*)

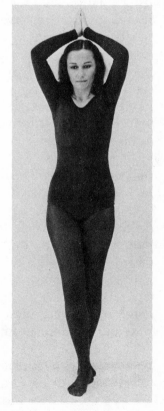

Foot in Front Pose

ulates vital organs in the lower part of the abdomen.

One substitute allowed for this exercise is the foot in front balancing pose: Bring right foot in front of left foot so that heel touches big toe and both feet are in a straight line. Arms are raised and palms joined above head. Eyes are closed. Pose should be maintained for at least 6 deliberate slow breaths.

Stretching and Twisting Poses

In chapter 8 on shaping the body, a number of *asanas* restoring suppleness were given. In the context of rebirth, the following seven *asanas* related to the human spine should be mastered as closely as possible:

EXERCISE 1: Forward-Stretching Pose *(Passimotasana)*
This exercise begins with one seated on a comfortable mat, both legs stretched forward. After exhaling breath, bend body forward, index fingers securing a good hold on big toes, while you bring head down to knees. Pose is completely mastered when you are capable of retaining this position while breathing without difficulty.

EXERCISE 2: Angular Pose *(Konasana)*
Seated with back and neck in a straight line, bring both heels close to the body, knees apart, again securing hold of big toes with the index fingers. Exhale. Then lean body slightly backward and stretch legs up and sideways at a 45-degree angle, straightening knees. Upon completely stretching both knees, retain pose with breath even and rhythmical for a minute or two.

EXERCISE 3: Pose of the Plough *(Halasana)*
Seated with back and neck in a straight line, bring legs over the head and again secure the big toes with

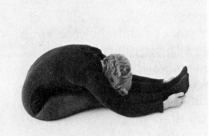

Forward-Stretching Pose
(*Passimotasana*)

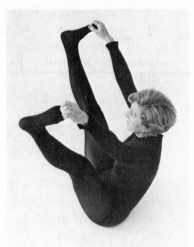

Angular Pose (*Konasana*)

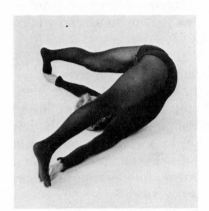

Pose of the Plough—
Holding Toes (*Halasana*)

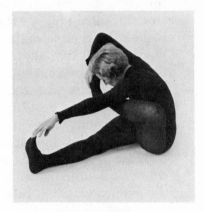

Pose of an Archer
(*Akarshana Dhaburasana*)

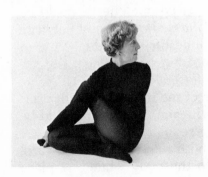

Modified Twist
(*Ardha-Matsyendrasana*)

the index finger. With the feet apart, maintain breath as in the two previous positions.

All three poses described above are united by the same principle: ability to breathe without difficulty in three different attitudes—stretched forward, balanced on the buttocks, and with the legs over the head. This is possible only in cases of correct bodily weight and suppleness. If the weight hasn't been adjusted or the body is still stiff, these are impossible to perform.

Another interesting aspect of this position is the following: It is believed that rhythmical breathing while holding the big toes with the index fingers locks the current of life force within the human body, nourishing and vitalizing every organ.

EXERCISE 4: Pose of an Archer
    Seated on a mat, both legs stretched forward, place the right foot on the other side of the left knee. Sitting straight, inhale fully. After complete exhalation, the left hand holds the toe of the right foot while the right hand holds the left foot and raises it with the aim of touching the point between the eyebrows. In the same manner, do the exercise with the legs reversed.

This pose is a beautiful and dynamic one, portraying the movement of the archer pulling the string of a bow. It is designed to limber up practically every joint of the body. It is said that the flow of cosmic energy could be consciously directed to the *Ajna* chakra, or point between the eyebrows, when the final gesture is made.

EXERCISE 5: Twist *(Ardha-Matsyendrasana)*
    The classical twist is one of the most important exercises to keep the spine healthy and mobile. It should be mastered and practiced on a regular basis.

Seated on the floor with both legs extended forward, bring the right heel close to the body while you place the left foot over the right knee. The left knee is then locked under the right armpit, with the right arm firmly holding the left ankle. Bring the left arm around the back. Upon complete exhalation, twist the body to the left, creating the same sensation of movement in each joint of the spinal column. The movement is repeated on the other side.

EXERCISE 6: Pose of a Dove *(Kapotha Asana)*

Seated on the floor with both feet at the right side, bend the knees. Raise the outside foot and hook it into the curve of the right elbow, while the hands are brought behind the head and the fingers interlaced. Pose and breath should be maintained without difficulty.

EXERCISE 7: Variation of *Yoga Mudra*

Seated in the free pose, bring the body forward until the forehead rests on the floor. Stretch both arms forward as far as possible, with palms resting on the floor. Unlike the *mudra* where the breath is retained to create pressure in the head, in this exercise the student is challenged to maintain the pose and rhythmical breath without difficulty.

Backward-Bending *Asanas*

Liberation of the body from stiffness can't be achieved without mastering the seven backward-bending *asanas*. Apart from limbering the spine in the reverse direction of the forward-stretching poses, those *asanas* stimulate the adrenal glands located at the top of the kidneys. They also tone up the roots of the spinal nerves and increase the flow of arterial blood to vital organs located in the lower abdomen.

EXERCISE 1: Cobra *(Bujangasana)*

Lying flat on the stomach with the toes stretched backward, place hands palms down beside the body with the fingertips at shoulder level. With inhalation, the body is pushed up and the small of the back arched as much as possible. Breath and pose are retained for a few seconds, and the body is then lowered to the original position while breath is exhaled. Practice 3–4 times with the mind concentrated on the region of the small of the back and on the thought of toning up the adrenal glands.

EXERCISE 2: Pose of the Bow *(Dhanurasana)*

Lying as before, raise legs with a good hold secured on both ankles. With inhalation, the body is raised up in the attitude of a bow, pose and breath retained as previously given. With exhalation, body is lowered. To be practiced 2–3 times.

EXERCISE 3: Half Bow *(Ardha-Dhanurasana)*

Lying as above, bend only the right leg, with a good grip secured on the right ankle with the right hand. The left arm is stretched forward. With inhalation, three parts of the body are raised: left arm, left leg, and right knee. The body is gracefully balanced in the attitude of the previous exercise with the left and right legs stretched. After practicing twice, reverse position of legs and arms.

EXERCISE 4: Pose of a Locust *(Salabhasana)*

Starting as above (flat on the stomach), bring arms alongside the body, fists closed. With inhalation, in a powerful and rather fast movement, raise both legs as high as possible, retaining pose and breath and returning to the original position with exhalation. 2–3 times.

EXERCISE 5: Pose of a Camel *(Ushtrasana)*

Balancing on the knees with knees slightly apart and hands in the attitude of prayer in front of the chest, inhale deeply and then lower body backward while exhaling until both hands are able to secure ankles. This gracefully arched pose should be maintained for a minute or two while breath is kept even and rhythmical.

EXERCISE 6: Pose of a Fish *(Matsyasana)*
Seated with the legs locked in the lotus position, slowly lower the body backward until the crown of the head rests on the floor. Knees should be pressed to the floor and arms placed underneath the neck. Breath is rhythmical and deep.
Apart from limbering up the spine, this pose is extremely beneficial for the neck and throat and upper part of the lungs, which are participating vigorously in the breathing process.

EXERCISE 7: Pose of the Wheel (Chakra *Asana*)
The pose of the wheel nourishes and stimulates all seven chakras of the body, hence the name chakra *asana.*
Lie on the back, with knees drawn up and feet as close to the body as possible. Hands are inverted and placed at both sides of the head. With inhalation, entire body is raised into the graceful position known in Western gymnastics as a bridge. The pose is maintained for 1–2 minutes; breath is rhythmical and deep.

Raised *Asanas*

Raised poses have a particular role in yoga training. They are skillfully designed to convey the sensation of lightness and strength, and if done on a regular basis, they are capable of checking the sensation of heaviness typical of older years, even if the weight of the body does not increase. Significantly, most raised poses have the names of birds or names suggesting lightness. Ultimate mastery of these poses includes the ability to retain them with

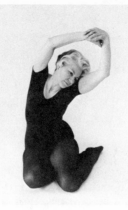

Pose of a Dove
(*Kapotha Asana*)

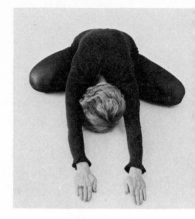

Cross-Legged pose—stretching
forward. Variation of *Yoga Mudra*

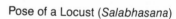

Pose of the Bow (*Dhanurasana*)

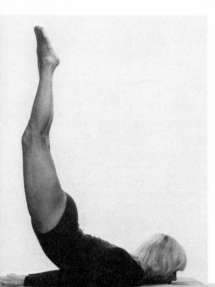

Pose of a Locust (*Salabhasana*)

Pose of a Locust—
Modified (*Ardha-Salabhasana*)

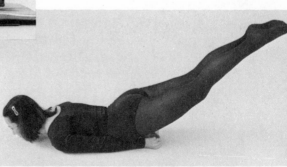

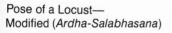

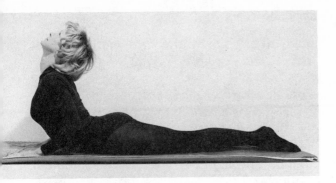

Cobra (*Bujangasana*)

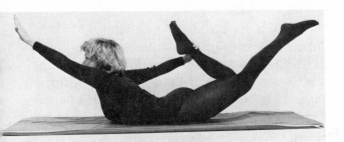

Half Bow (*Ardha-Dhanurasana*)

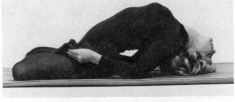

Pose of a Fish (*Matsyasana*)

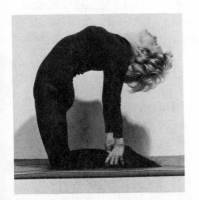

Pose of a Camel (*Ushtrasana*)

Pose of the Wheel (Chakra *Asana*)

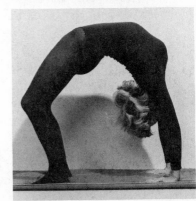

ease long enough to say slowly the most famous of all mantras: *om ma ne pad me hum.*[3]

EXERCISE 1: Pose of a Bird *(Kavasana)*
    Squatting, place arms between the knees, palms resting on the floor. With inhalation, the body is moved forward until knees rest on top of the elbows while feet are stretched out and brought together, forming the tail of the bird. Position and breath are retained for 6 heartbeats, then body is lowered to original position. Exhale. Repeat exercise.

EXERCISE 2: Pose of a Raven
    Instead of placing arms inside the knees, bring knees together and place arms at the side of knees. The right arm is brought to the outside of the left knee; as in the bird pose, the bent leg is pressed against the arm beside it, which takes the weight of the body. During the final attitude, breath is retained. After performing the right aspect, repeat with the left.

EXERCISE 3: Pose of a Floating Cloud
    This pose is also known as the pose of eight curves. Sitting comfortably on your exercise mat, with back and neck in a straight line, cross the ankles, with knees slightly bent. Insert your right arm (or stronger arm) between the thighs, and lock the right thigh against the right elbow, which is bent. The left arm is in line with the right, with both palms flat on the floor. Inhale and raise your hips off the floor, leaving the feet still in contact with the floor. Then raise your feet off the floor, so that the body, supported by the hands, is clear of the floor and parallel to it, floating above it as a cloud. The whole body is interlocked in such a way that the right thigh rests

    3. "Hail the jewel in the lotus flower."

on the right elbow and the left foot is locked with the right foot. In the beginning, the position is held for only a few seconds, gradually increasing the duration to a few minutes. When the pose is fully mastered it should be maintained without difficulty while breathing is rhythmical. It should also be practiced using the left or weaker arm as a support.

Apart from the sensation of lightness, the sensation of accentuated bodily awareness is increased by the practice of this *asana,* in which each part of the body coordinates with the other in a balanced way. Due to the slight curvature of the spine and tension in the back muscles, nervous centers along the spinal cord are supplied with an extra flow of arterial blood, toned up, and stimulated.

EXERCISE 4: Raised Lotus

A classical raised pose of three yogas. Seated on an exercise mat, lock legs in a lotus position, place hands at the sides of the body, palms on floor. With inhalation, raise the entire body clear of the floor.

The *Manipura* chakra, or solar plexus, gets an extra flow of arterial blood during this posture; the entire system is toned up and stimulated.

EXERCISE 5: Pose of a Crane

Seated on the floor, raise the right leg and lock it over the right elbow while the palms of both hands rest on the floor. The left leg is stretched forward. With inhalation, raise the body clear of the floor, and retain the position for the same time as in previous exercises. Then repeat the pose, using left arm and left leg.

EXERCISE 6: Pose of a Peacock *(Mayurasana)*

One of the most graceful raised poses is the pose of the peacock, in which the entire body, while stretched

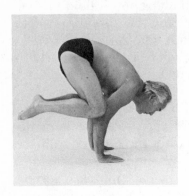

Pose of a Bird (*Kavasana*)

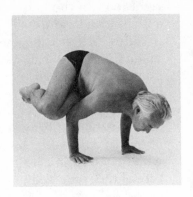

Pose of a Raven (*Kavasana*)

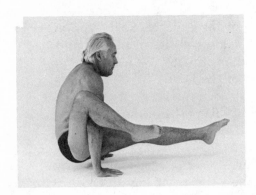

Pose of a Crane

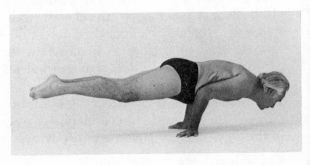

Pose of a Peacock (*Mayurasana*)

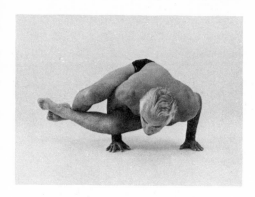

Pose of a Floating Cloud
(Eight Curves) (*Astha Vakrasana*)

Raised Lotus
(*Utthita Padmasana*)

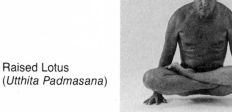

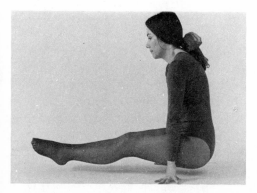

Finger Pose

parallel to the floor with face down, is supported by arms bent at the elbows and palms down on the floor. The support is actually on the elbows. This position can be performed in two different ways. The way suggested to beginners is to stretch out, face downward, with the upper part of the body raised to allow the elbows to be placed underneath the abdomen as the hands are placed palms downward on the floor with the fingers toward the feet. Toes are still on the floor, so the entire body is supported by palms and toes (which in itself is known as the pose of the duck). The full peacock pose occurs when the toes are raised off the floor and the entire body is resting on the elbows, supported by the palms. Breath is retained and held long enough as in the previous exercises to say the mantra.

The more demanding way to do it is to start from a kneeling position with the knees apart and hands on the ground between them, fingers pointing toward the toes. Elbows are tightly pressed to the abdomen, and legs are slowly stretched like a peacock tail parallel to the floor.

An important aspect of this position is the pressure of the elbows in the region of the solar plexus, which tones up and charges this important center with extra energy.

EXERCISE 7: Finger Pose

The ultimate test of bodily strength in relationship to weight, as well as a test of general condition, is the finger pose. Seated on the floor with the legs outstretched, place hands (with fingers spread) at each side of the body. With inhalation, raise the entire body clear off the floor, so the weight of the body is supported by the fingertips. Duration of this position is the same as above. Breath is exhaled and body is lowered to original position.

In the tradition of Taoist yoga, prior to practicing this

position, a gentle breath is practiced for a few minutes, as it is believed that this contributes to the sensation of lightness.

This rather demanding pose can be done without difficulty by a young person in good physical condition, but the idea is to retain or regain the ability to do it as easily in your senior years as in youth.

Seven Inverted *Asanas*

The inverted positions are the most important bodily positions in terms of their influence on the body condition. They are designed to improve circulation, to counteract the detrimental effects of gravitational pull by sending an extra flow of arterial blood to the upper body, especially the head. They stimulate the endocrine glands, help to prevent varicose veins, and readjust vital organs of the abdomen that may have become displaced.

They have to be practiced on a regular basis. Being static positions, they should always be supported by breath control and constructive thinking. The amount of time spent in each of these positions depends on the individual; one should practice each pose as long as is comfortable. It is important to consult "the inner guru" regarding the length of time to hold any given exercise. One should come down slowly and rest after each position before starting the next one. A soft, comfortable mat should be used for all these *asanas*.

EXERCISE 1: Shoulder Stand *(Sarvangasana)*
This exercise is considered to be the second most powerful of all the bodily poses, surpassed only by the headstand in its beneficial effects on the body.

Lying flat on a mat, raise legs, hips, and torso slowly

until the chin becomes tightly pressed to the chest and the whole body assumes a vertical position. Hands support the back, eyes are closed, breath is deep and rhythmical. In the tradition I learned, the tip of the tongue touches the soft palate in a gesture known as *manduka mudra (frog mudra)*. The student is instructed to retain this *mudra* until the pleasant sensation of sweetness is experienced on the tip of the tongue.

A reference in ancient treatises to this particular practice is descriptive of its effects: "A wise yogi who drinks daily the nectar of the thousand-petaled lotus is free from diseases, endowed with longevity, possesses a luminous body, and conquers the ravages of old age. Indeed, he can conquer death itself." Discussing this enigmatic saying with teachers in the East, I came to the conclusion that a remarkable biochemical process takes place in the human body while one is engaged in this *asana*. In the neck there is a nest of very important glands: the thyroid, parathyroid, tonsils, and saliva glands. Due to the position of the chin and the extra flow of arterial blood, those glands become stimulated. The pituitary and the pineal glands in the brain are also stimulated. The "drop of the thousand-petaled lotus" in my opinion is nothing else but the combined secretions of all these glands. The secretions join in the throat almost as in an alchemical laboratory to create an elixir of life. If it is true that "we are as young as our glands," then this is a key exercise to keep us young. Regular stimulation of the endocrine glands is one of the answers to the problem of aging and to prolonging creative life.

The psychosomatic effect of constructive thinking is also an important part of this practice, while deep and rhythmical breathing increases the flow of cosmic energy, or *prana*, into the system.

EXERCISE 2: Inverted Gesture *(Viparetha Karani)*

Closely resembling the previous position is the pose known as the half shoulder stand to the Western student. It is executed in practically the same manner as the pose described above, but instead of going up all the way, only half of the back is raised, leaving the shoulder blades still in contact with the floor. The hands support the hips (chin is not pressed to chest), and more pressure is experienced by the elbows supporting the weight of hips and trunk. The eyes are closed, and breath is deep and rhythmical as in the previous position.

Due to the inverted attitude of the legs, hips, and abdominal region, as well as to the pressure on the elbows, an extensive flow of arterial blood is directed to the head, toning up and stimulating the skin of the face as well as the facial tissues, and thus preventing the face from going through the deterioration normally associated with aging. The student is instructed to evoke an image of himself youthful and unchangeable, and to project this image into the future. In a way, he is engaged in a session of self-hypnosis while practicing this position, by reprogramming his psyche to help the body remain younger longer.

EXERCISE 3: Pose of Longevity

The Taoist tradition teaches an inverted pose known also as the pose of tranquility. Lying on the back, raise legs, hips, and trunk slowly and point over the head at a 45-degree angle. At the same time, both arms are raised up, catching the legs at the knees and bringing the knees to rest on the hands. It is important to achieve a steady position. The body is balanced on the shoulders, with the raised arms supporting the weight of the legs and thus relieving much pressure from the spine. The chin is tightly pressed to the chest, and a certain amount of

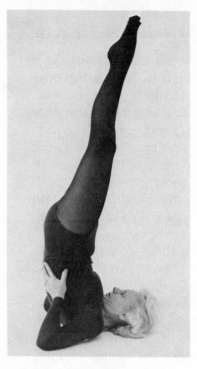

Shoulder Stand (*Sarvangasana*)

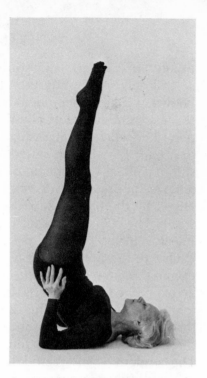

Inverted Gesture (*Viparetha Karani*)

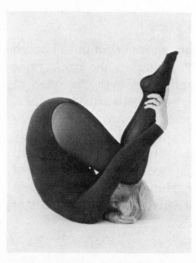

Yin/Yang Pose (Taoist Yoga)

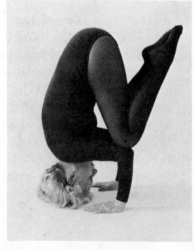

Half Headstand Pose
(*Ardha-Shirshasana*)

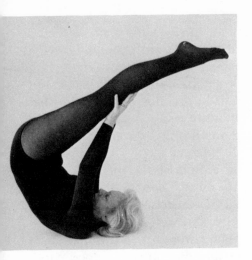

Pose of Longevity (Tranquillity) (Taoist Yoga)

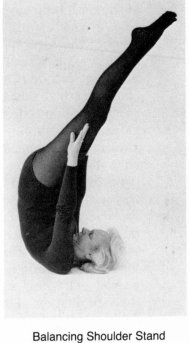

Balancing Shoulder Stand

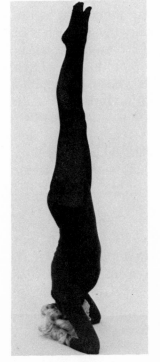

Headstand (*Shirshasana*)

pressure is experienced at the back of the neck. Looking at the position from the side, it resembles a triangle, one side of which is the back, another the raised arms, and another the legs. With a little practice, the position becomes very easy and pleasant to retain. As in all inverted positions, it should be retained only as long as comfortable. Breath should be rhythmical.

The position is designed to nourish the medulla oblongata, or little brain, at the lower part of the skull. An ancient claim suggests that this exercise can give freedom from disease, lasting energy, and well-being, and can expand one's life to 150 years through the stimulation of this organ by the extensive flow of nourishing blood. Modern scientific discoveries verify this claim almost to the point. As I mentioned earlier, the latest research of gerontologists suggests that the medulla may be responsible for manufacturing a "youth hormone," but as the years pass, it gets progressively lazier. It has been suggested that stimulation of this organ by mild electrical shock could result in a longer period of production of this youth hormone. Some scientists have voiced the opinion that through such measures human life indeed could be prolonged up to 150 years.

Another aspect of this position is that it puts the entire nervous system in a state of balanced peace and tranquility and helps to improve the quality of sleep and to combat insomnia.

EXERCISE 4: Balancing Shoulder Stand

Legs, hips, and trunk are raised in very much the same manner as in the previous position, but the aim of the practicer here is to have his body as vertical as possible while arms are also raised straight up at the sides of the body.

In some old treatises of Taoist yoga, I found it mentioned that this position stimulates the pineal gland, symbolically referred to as the "third eye," an organ of the higher faculty of human makeup. The position does change the entire circulation, in the arms as well as in the rest of the body. In other inverted poses, the arms are used for supporting or balancing the body.

EXERCISE 5: Yin/Yang Pose

Another inverted pose of Chinese yoga. After the body is raised straight up as in the balancing shoulder stand described previously, the legs are slowly lowered, both knees coming to rest on the forehead, while toes are pointed straight up. To complete the pose, the ankles are held by the hands. Looking at the position from the side, one with some imagination could recognize the ancient yin/yang sign of male and female principles encircled by Tao.

Claims related to this position are quite extraordinary. I touched on them in chapter 1 about physical changes in the process of aging. Mastery and regular practice of this position leads to perfect balance of male and female principles within. It arrests the phenomenon of imbalance in the hormones when the aging man in some cases develops female characteristics and vice versa.

EXERCISE 6: Half Headstand Pose, or Tripod Pose

This is a preparatory pose for the complete headstand position. The student starts to learn it by kneeling on the mat, placing the crown of the head on the mat. The palms of the hands form two sides of a triangle, with the head as the apex. Next, the knees are raised off the floor and the practicer walks a few little steps toward his head, then places right and left knees respectively on top of the right and left elbows. Duration of practice and breathing are the same as in all inverted poses described previously.

EXERCISE 7: Headstand *(Shirshasana)*

Sometimes known as the skull gesture, this exercise is known in yogic tradition as the king of all bodily poses. It has the most profound effect on the entire body, changing blood circulation polarity and the magnetic current in the body. It also counteracts gravitational pull, helping to correct displacement of organs. Its most important effect is to nourish the brain with a supply of arterial blood, thus toning up the pineal and pituitary glands. In the Indian tradition, the head position delays aging, prevents and cures varicose veins, improves memory and concentration, and cures a great number of other physical and mental maladies. It has to be practiced with great caution and with the guidance of an experienced teacher. During this practice, one should listen to the voice of "the guru within" more carefully than in any of the other poses, so that you know when to terminate it.

The headstand is completely forbidden in cases of hypertension, weak eye capillaries (bloodshot eyes), and chronic afflictions of the ears. Many teachers do not encourage the practice of the headstand by people over sixty, while some suggest age fifty as a limit. In my experience, people who start to practice the head posture in their youth or in middle life, who enjoy good health and are free from arteriosclerosis, can successfully and beneficially practice this position even at the age of seventy-five.

The position should never be practiced on a full stomach or in a state of mental anguish or depression. Morning and evening are the best times for practicing this position.

The exercise also starts from the kneeling position. This time, the fingers are interlaced and placed firmly on the mat, thumbs on top, forming a little enclosure where the crown of the head is put while the back of the head is held by interlaced fingers. Knees are raised and the student walks, as in the previous pose, toward his head until the trunk of his body is quite vertical. Toes are slowly lifted off the floor, and the body is gradually unfolded into a vertical position, balancing on the crown of the head and forearms. The student keeps his body very straight, eliminating as much as possible an arch in the small of the back which puts unnecessary pressure on this part of the spine. It is very important to start with only a few seconds and gradually build the duration of the pose to a few minutes, but always retaining it only as long as is comfortable. Establish rhythmical breath.

Seven Meditations

1. Meditation on Rebirth

Oh, spring without end, with boundaries. . . .
—Alexander Blok

The essential self or spirit in each of us is eternally youthful. Through meditation we can experience vividly that part of ourselves which is like an eternal spring. This acknowledgment of a youthful self within is very important in delaying the aging process.

We know that the aging process can be accelerated by thinking ourselves old. If thought processes can trigger biological responses to accelerate aging, then the process must also work in the other direction. Regular meditation on the youthful self within will help us to express that self in a more radiant way.

The person who seriously desires to achieve rebirth should make a commitment through meditation to the success of his venture. One's first theme for meditation should be an image of a younger, healthier, and more enlightened self.

Seated comfortably in a meditative pose, close your eyes and try to imagine in detail how you would look and feel if you were at the peak of health, vitality, suppleness, attractiveness, and good spirits. Once the image becomes clear to you, identify yourself with that ideal person. Enjoy the pleasure of a graceful shape and radiant looks, of unencumbered and supple movement, or positive expectations from work, love, and play. Savor these sensations. Dedicate yourself to being born again.

This meditation should be practiced regularly until you no longer feel a need for it, when your psyche has readjusted so that you know without doubt that you can keep your commitment to the program because you have fully realized the possibility for the likelihood of attaining renewal.

2. Meditation on the Body

> This body is given to me—so unique, so totally mine. What can I do with it?
>
> —O. Mandelshtam

The physical body with its five senses is *our way of being in the world.* One cannot overemphasize the importance of taking care of its needs and in turn experiencing its well-being.

One of the main problems of modern Western man— and the cause of many physical maladies—is the loss of body consciousness through sedentary and cerebral occupations. In such a cultural condition, the body becomes an instrument driven by the mind into mechanical servitude. After committing yourself to rebirth, your next step should be to become acquainted with your body and to reach a higher plane of bodily awareness. If we conceive of the body as a temple of the living spirit (a cornerstone of both Eastern and Western thought), then we behave toward it with proper reverence.

Begin this meditation by closing your eyes, breathing deeply, and projecting your consciousness outside your body in order to obtain a detached view. Then allow the mind's eye to look inward. Try to acquire a new look at yourself as if from inside the body. By focusing attention exclusively on the physical self, we can acquire knowledge and sensitivity regarding the body's functioning.

The person only vaguely aware of the inner structure of his body may need to review information pertinent to his biology in order to visualize his separate parts with clarity. Needless to say, the visualization of these parts is only the beginning. The important task is to develop a sensitivity to each part as an entity with its own needs.

Once I discussed meditation on the physical body with my Chinese master. Among other things I asked him whether he had ever been to a doctor. He opened his eyes wide and for quite some time looked at me in true amazement. Then, deliberately choosing his words, he told me, "Why should I consult a doctor? Who knows my body better than myself? The finest specialists from every corner of the world could examine me—they still would not do it better than I can do it myself. I know my body. I have dwelled in it many years. I know it better and more intimately than I know this ashram where I have lived many years. It is the home of my spirit—my psyche—and I know it from within in such a manner that no other person could equal. When my time comes to depart into a different world, I will do it in the traditional way, with dignity and without remorse. After all, Buddha died, Christ died, and I will die, too. While I am here I will attend to my body's needs."

He was an elderly man at that time, but he possessed excellent health, abundance of energy, and a youthful and ever inquisitive spirit. How wonderful if each of us can become our own physician!

The proper attitude for this kind of meditation is to suspend for a time the despotism of the intellect. Inquire humbly of one body part at a time what its condition is and what it needs. Listen receptively, and you may be surprised at the response. I have known many succinct answers to occur to the mind's ear under those circumstances. They may be very simple: Shoulders may need rubbing; arms may need more diverse activity; hands may need to make something, the chest may need to be thrust forward more often; the waist may need to show more clearly; the abdomen may want to be felt more definitely as the center of one's body; hips may want to swing more freely or to support the body more; genitals may be over- or underemployed; thighs may want to move more gracefully; feet may need to be more in touch with nature. Proceeding inwardly, the brain may need more stimulation; the ears may need to listen more often; the "inner ear" may need to be opened; the nasal passages and throat may feel abused; the lungs may need greater expansion; the heart may want you to adjust your diet so that it can function more efficiently. These examples will give you some idea of the possibilities in a dialogue with the parts of the body.

Developing a dialogue with one's bodily parts can lead to benevolent mastery over bodily functions. This harmony, in turn, will lead to an extension of health and longevity.

3. Meditation on the Instinctive Mind

Millions of cell minds are like millions of warriors. Learn to lead them and you will win all battles.

—Michael Volin

There are two mainstreams of modern thought on the causes of aging. One is represented by Leonard Hayflick of Stanford University, who believes that each cell contains in its genetic program a predetermined life span and that it dies on schedule after a certain number of divisions (generally enough to permit the individual to grow to maturity, procreate, and raise children to the age of procreation). For Hayflick, the biological clock is in each cell. Another point of view is represented by W. D. Denckla, who believes that the clock of aging is in the brain and that aging is governed by the flow of hormones to body cells.

The most advanced research in gerontology clearly shows a correspondence between ancient esoteric knowledge and modern science. Yoga philosophy teaches that each cell of the body contains its own consciousness and can communicate directly with the governing intelligence of the mind. The mind has direct access to information needed for the health of the body's infinitesimal parts. This cell consciousness is referred to in yoga as the "instinctive mind," or "body wisdom."

The yoga point of view about aging is supported by Denckla's research into the importance of the brain in controlling aging. For centuries, yogis have practiced inverted postures to stimulate the pituitary and pineal glands, thus insuring a healthy flow of hormones to cells of the body. They have also practiced meditations to gain conscious control over the millions of instinctive minds in the body, thereby significantly influencing the health of the body through prevention of disease and rapid healing wherever disease and wounds occur.

After carefully considering both scientific points of view about aging and comparing them to what I have learned from yoga, my point of view is this: If the cells are individually programmed by nature to die at a specific time, the conscious mind, through meditation, can reprogram them to live longer. This leads us to the theme of our meditation on the instinctive mind. This meditation is given in three phases.

1. Seated in a meditative posture, breathing deeply and rhythmically, spend some time becoming aware of your body's cellular composition and concentrating on the idea that each cell has its own consciousness. After you are fully aware of the channel of communication between the conscious mind and the instinctive mind, practice the goodwill breath of the yogi, in which you direct *prana* supported by goodwill to every living cell of the body while you exhale each breath.

   In this exercise, millions of body cells can be stimulated by cosmic energy and inspiring thought. Regular practice of this exercise is believed to lead to restorative and recuperative powers as the cells begin to respond to the benevolent influence of the conscious mind.

2. Yoga teaches that another aspect of aging occurs when cells die because they have become clogged with impurities. We can also practice meditation to purify the cells of our bodies. Through direct contact with the instinctive mind we can accelerate the mechanisms in charge of the purification of cells by stimulating each cell to more vigorous activity with each breath.

3. In the third phase of this meditation you can attempt to influence the very nucleus of your body cells by taking control of the instinctive mind. After practicing the goodwill breath and the breath for purification of cells, speak to the cells with your mind's voice: *You may be programmed to die. But you vibrate on an instinctive level. I vibrate on a higher level. I will reprogram you. You are going to live in good health until I am ready to die.*

The metaphysical tradition of the East teaches that the body cells eventually respond to and obey the suggestions of the governing mind, which exercises the constructive power of thought. It further teaches that in the golden age of humankind, human intelligence possessed absolute power to heal, recharge, and rejuvenate the body. In the dark age that followed, this power was lost. Reminders of it can be found in the property of some lower animals to grow new limbs, the power having been taken from human beings.

Perhaps the reader is familiar with the work of Edgar Cayce, the American "sleeping prophet" who reportedly was able to do "readings," or diagnoses, of illnesses by entering with his mind's eye the body of a person with physical impairments. The story of his traveling through a person's body with his mind's eye while Cayce was in a trance until he found the diseased spot parallels what I am suggesting here about what each of us can do for ourselves if we become sufficiently sensitive to the inner workings of our bodies. This process may still sound alien to the Westerner's perception, but it is a long accepted practice in the Eastern metaphysical tradition of paying attention to the instinctive mind, or body wisdom. This meditation offers us a way to become our own physician, at least to a much greater degree than most of us are aware.

4. Meditation on Personal Time

> In eternity, time stands still. By moving closer to the eternity within you, you are slowing down your personal time.
> —Michael Volin

Meditation on the movement of time within is one of the practices of Taoist yoga that is designed to slow the aging process.

Modern medical experience has shown us that anxiety, stress, and trauma greatly accelerate the aging process in some mysterious way, as if these nervous and emotional diseases cause the biological clock to go haywire. We also know that one physiological manifestation of these diseases is shallow breathing. Deep breathing exercises often are recommended as a means of calming anxiety or simple stress.

This meditation, in which we direct the beam of the perceiving consciousness to the mysterious passage of time within, begins with deep and rhythmical breathing to bring about tranquility of mind and body. When that state is achieved, turn your mind's eye to the "spaceless space" within, the region of the middle of the chest corresponding to the *Anahata* chakra. Concentrate on becoming aware of the movement of time within yourself. If you concentrate long enough you will become aware of that movement. It will be a nonintellectual experience in which you suddenly know, as direct truth, your own rhythm of time.

In my own experience, the realization of personal time flow appeared as a gray stream coming from nowhere and flowing nowhere, but mercilessly moving through my inner space. It was again like a large wheel that set other smaller wheels in motion, relentlessly wearing down and destroying the molecules of my material existence. I was so moved by this insight that I exerted all my powers against this involuntary passage of time through my space. The meditation then brought me to the spontaneous recognition that I was capable of slowing the passage of time. When that realization struck me, I behaved with such ecstatic joy that I began to dance. My friends who were meditating with me thought me mad until I calmed down and told them what had happened.

Once you have achieved this dual awareness of your own personal time and your capability to slow down its rhythm, you can start to experiment with your breathing. Be aware that just as rapid and uneven breathing accelerates your time clock, slow and rhythmical breathing will bring it under control. Be conscious that the intrusion of disturbing thoughts and anxieties causes you to lose control of your breathing and of time. Act on the principle that by exercising your own free will you can influence the passage of time within yourself. Experiment with your breathing until you are convinced that while you are in this tranquil inner space you are in touch with eternity, where there is no time as we know it.

In this way, meditation on personal time brings one close to one of the great mysteries of life, the mystery of time. We have various ways and means to track time: the changes from day to night as the earth rotates around its axis; the changes from season to season, from year to year. These ways of measuring time actually tell us little about time itself. I don't propose to try to solve the mystery of time here, but I would like to share with you my belief that regular experience of that sense of eternity through meditation contributes to one's inner strength and gives one the power to challenge time.

As you move deeper into your own "spaceless space" you realize that you are moving deeper into eternity. Once you have entered this space, you can return to it whenever you need a retreat—a place to calm yourself, allowing your psyche to adjust to the shocks and stresses that time brings to us all in our outer lives. You can return to it regularly as a preventive measure against ill health and aging.

5. Meditation on the Seed of Immortality in the Breath

In the chapters on breathing, I have already suggested how one can recognize the vital significance of breath and begin to harness cosmic energy, or *prana,* through breathing exercises, many of which include concentration on various parts of the body as *prana* is directed to them. I cannot overemphasize the value of realizing that breath not only animates and charges the body with vitality; it is also our most intimate experience with the cosmos. By drawing breath into our bodies, we partake of the force that animates all the creatures in the universe and makes possible the growth of all living things.

Our Western orientation leads us to think of all living creatures as separate entities, and in a sense, of course, we are. However, it is strangely satisfying to realize that all living creation is one whole, the separate parts of which are linked by their relation to air. That vital link can be experienced through meditation on breathing, particularly the exercise described earlier in which we try to identify with our breath, to pass out of "normal" consciousness into a superconsciousness which makes us feel at one with the cosmos.

This Eastern form of meditation strikingly resembles the teachings of the Greek philosopher Anaximander, who taught the doctrine of cosmic breath *(pneuma),* which animates the entire universe in the same manner as the individual breath animates each of us.

Meditation on the seed of immortality in the breath is directly related to challenging time. Seated in a meditative posture, breathing deeply and rhythmically, concentrate on the subtle moment when incoming breath becomes outgoing breath. As I mentioned in chapter 5 on breathing exercises, in the metaphysical tradition the incoming breath symbolizes life and the outgoing breath symbolizes death. The moment when the incoming breath becomes the outgoing breath is known as the point of immortality. Meditation on this point, or seed, brings one closer and closer to the realization of the immortality of one's essential self. This realization contributes greatly to mental serenity and thus to general well-being.

6. Meditation on Personal Immortality

What did your face look like before your parents were born?

—Zen koan

For this meditation I would like to share with you another personal experience. In the practices of Zen Buddhism, koans (statements or questions that defy intellectual interpretation) are used for meditation. Once I was seated before my master, who gave me the koan, "What did your face look like before your parents were born?" Immediately, my intellect rebelled and I could not conceal my amazement. The master sternly repeated the koan and then circled me like an eagle, fortifying something deep within me by repeating this koan again and again. Then there was a long silence, as if it were known to my master that I was ready to enter a higher plane of consciousness, and in this long silence I realized as direct truth that I did have a face—in fact, many faces, thousands—before my parents were born. I knew without doubt that my present birth was not the first and only one; I was born into the world many times before.

Later on, when acquainted with the philosophy of Schopenhauer, I found further confirmation of my experience with the koan. He stated that if he were asked by an Asian man for a definition of Europe, he would tell him that Europe is the part of the world where exists the preposterous belief that our birth into this life is the first, only, and final one. Through the meditation on this koan, I discovered for myself the mysterious transcendental truth of the great law of reincarnation and the immortality of my spirit. I believe that one who meditates on this koan might achieve a similar revelation.

7. Meditation on Cosmic Unity

Everything is in me and I am in everything.

—F. Tutcheff

Anyone who ever observed a living cell under the microscope is struck by the thought that the cell is expanding and contracting as if it were breathing. A long time before electronic microscopes were invented, the ancients were aware of this phenomenon. They called it vibration, the last indivisible part of matter. They also taught that this expansion and contraction of the cell corresponds remarkably to the expansion and contraction of the entire universe. In some incredible way this idea brings us closer to another great mystery of the universe, the correspondence of microcosm and macrocosm.

Seated in a meditative posture, concentrate first on the rhythm of your breath, then on that same rhythm as inherent in each of your bodily cells. Allow your perceptions then to move outward in expanded motion until you become aware of this vibratory motion in the world, in the universe. Continue the meditation as you come closer and closer to a realization of belonging to an intricate cosmic structure, the parts of which vibrate simultaneously with the life force. This realization fortifies the personal knowledge of immortality and greatly contributes to inner strength and serenity, two of the main factors in health and longevity.

Glossary

Advasana: Pose of relaxation in the prone position.

Ajna chakra: In Indian yoga, the psychic center located between the eyebrows commonly identified with the third eye, corresponding with the pineal gland accepted as the dormant organ of the higher faculty of man.

Anahata chakra: In Indian yoga, the psychic center corresponding with the cardiac plexus, the first of the higher-level chakras where more refined feelings are experienced.

Ananda: Means "perfect bliss."

Apana: Vital energy related to excretory power of the body.

Aparoksha: Instantaneously obtained truth. Enlightenment.

Ardha-Dhanurasana: Exercise known also as half bow pose or flying fish pose.

Ardha-Matsyendrasana: Exercise known also as spinal half twist.

Asana: Sanskrit for "bodily pose."

Ashram: In the East, a retreat where yoga meditation and associated disciplines are practiced.

Ashvini mudra: Exercise involving contraction of the rectal muscles.

Astral body: In the Eastern metaphysical tradition, the third of seven body compositions of human makeup.

Aura: The emanation of the second or ethereal body in the Eastern metaphysical tradition which extends beyond the boundaries of the physical body and which can be seen by people sensitive to nonphysical manifestations.

Avatar: A highly evolved being who descends into human form.

Avatara yoga: The highest form of yoga, related to secret doctrines of yoga and not mentioned in traditional treatises. A form of yoga which leads to complete development, including the arresting of the aging process in the body.

Bandha: Sanskrit for "lock." In yoga, it refers to various techniques such as chin lock, contraction of rectal muscles, and drawing in of the abdomen.

Bhakti yoga: In India, the yoga of religious devotion.

Bhastrika (Blacksmith Bellows): One of the breath controls designed to oxygenate the bloodstream.

Bhramari (Bee): A breath control producing a humming sound not unlike the sound of a bee. Often related to the mantra of health, which creates beneficial vibrations throughout the body.

Bhunamanasana: A forward-stretching pose that develops limberness of the spine and locks vital energy within the system.

Blok, Alexander (1880–1921): Major poet of the silver age of Russian poetry.

Body sculpting: A process of shaping the body to one's own satisfaction by following a carefully designed program of muscle-toning exercises.

Body wisdom: A concept in Indian yoga of the body having the ability to communicate essential information about its needs through the medium of the instinctive mind.

Bordo: In the Tibetan tradition, the art of dying.

Brahma chakra (thousand-petaled lotus): The highest psychic center, it is generally accepted to represent the upper cortex of the brain.

Buddha, Gautama or Gotama: The founder of the religion called Buddhism. An Indian prince who lived circa 500 B.C. He abandoned his aristocratic wealth and position to seek enlightenment, which he received during prolonged meditation.

Buddha: An enlightened person who experiences cosmic realization.

Buddhism: A religion based on the teachings of Buddha which spread throughout India, China, Japan, and Tibet, embracing millions of followers.

Bujangasana (Cobra): One of the backward-bending postures that develops suppleness of the spine. Beneficial for organs in the lower abdomen.

Chadakasha space: "Spaceless space" within, thought to be located in the area of the cardiac plexus, or *Anahata* chakra.

Chakras: In Indian thought, the seven psychic centers in the human makeup (the yogic anatomy of the subtle body). They correspond, to a certain extent, with nervous centers of the physical body. From the base, they are (1) *Muladara,* (2) *Svadisthana,* (3) *Manipura,* (4) *Anahata,* (5) *Vishuddha,* (6) *Ajna,* (7) *Brahma.*

Chakra asana (Pose of the Wheel): This backward-bending pose stimulates all seven chakras, hence its name. It is also called the bridge pose in the West.

Chi: Chinese name for cosmic energy *(prana).*

Chigoon: Chinese healing breath.

Chinese yoga: Variation of Indian yoga with emphasis on longevity. Originated in India and introduced to China around the second century A.D.

Chuang-tzu: Chinese philosopher—followed Lao-tzu and developed Taoism.

Cosmic consciousness: Highest possible state of awareness. Identification of individual spirit with the spirit of the universe.

Dhanurasana (Pose of the Bow): This backward-bending pose develops suppleness of the spine.

Dharana: Concentration.

Dhyana: Meditation.

Dumo: The Tibetan art of creating psychic heat in which one dresses oneself in the warm cloth of his breath.

Ekapadasana: One of the balancing poses.

Garudasana (Pose of an Eagle): A balancing pose that helps to develop concentration as well.

Gomukhasana (Cow Head Pose): This stretching exercise develops suppleness of the shoulders and arms.

Guru: Spiritual teacher. It is said that there are three gurus for every person: (1) God, (2) the inner guru, and (3) one's spiritual guide in the outer world.

"Ha" breath: Cleansing breath that resembles a sigh of relief.

Halasana (Pose of the Plough): A stretching pose that leads to suppleness of the spine and tones up roots of spinal nerves, as well as thyroid and parathyroid glands.

Hatha yoga: In India, a physical yoga sometimes described as "reintegration through bodily strength."

Hathayoga Pradipika: One of the ancient Indian treatises on physical yoga.

Higher mind: An Eastern concept of a human faculty that is linked to cosmic consciousness and partakes of a universal wisdom, arrived at by intuition rather than rational thought processes.

Holistic health: Total health of body, mind, and soul.

Ida: In Indian yoga a nervous-psychic channel located in the left nostril and running alongside the spine to the *Muladara* chakra.

Incarnation: The embodiment of spirit, or the present life of an individual.

Indian yoga: The oldest of yogas. According to some schools of thought, Indian yoga could be 5,000 years old. Indian yoga takes a variety of paths, several of which are described herein.

Inner guru: A combination of common sense and intuition that manifests itself as an inner voice.

Instinctive mind: Mind locked in the cells of the body.

Intuition: A faculty of the higher mind in yogic thought—the perceiving power of the mind which leaps beyond the rational thought process to arrive spontaneously at insight.

Jalandhara bandha (Chin Lock): One of the techniques used in breath control and other exercises designed to prevent the escape of life force from the body.

Jharandasamhita: An ancient treatise on yoga postures and breathing.

Jnana yoga: In India, a yoga that involves re-integration through accumulation of wisdom and knowledge.

Ka: Life force in Egyptian tradition comparable to *chi* in Chinese thought or *Prana* in Indian tradition.

Kapotha asana (Pose of a Dove): A stretching pose in the cycle of limbering exercises.

Karma: In Indian thought, karma refers to the universal law of cause and effect, carried over from one lifetime to the next; karma plays a prominent part in the theory of reincarnation.

Karma yoga: In India, a yoga which follows a path of unselfish action.

Kavasana (Pose of a Bird): A raised pose designed to convey the sensation of lightness.

Kechari mudra: An unusual technique for bringing the body into a state resembling hibernation. It begins by pulling on the tongue with the fingers for many weeks to lengthen it. Then, before sleeping, the tongue is rolled backward, closing the glottis. This results in a considerable slowing of the metabolic rate, heartbeat, and blood pressure. Not recommended for the uninitiated.

Kirlian photography: A photographic technique discovered in Russia by Kirlian, using the principle of sensitive photo plates to record emanations from human fingertips, from leaves of trees, plants, and the like.

Koan: A technique of the Zen school of meditation: specially constructed sentences that defy intellectual interpretation and that are subjects for meditation.

Kumbhaka: Retention of full breath or emptiness between inhalation and exhalation.

Kundalini: A form of yoga dealing with the awakening of kundalini, or latent power, within human makeup. This power is symbolized as a snake coiled 3½ times around the base of the spine. Should only be practiced under an experienced guru.

Lama: A monk in Tibetan tradition.

Lamaseries: Tibetan monastic retreats.

Lao-tzu: Chinese philosopher said to have lived about 500 B.C. Founder of Taoism.

Maha: Means "great." One of the most important *mudras* involving retention of breath in a forward-stretched attitude is *Maha mudra.*

Mahavedha: *Mudra* of "great piercing." Technique involves striking the lower torso on the floor while seated in the lotus posture. Said to cause *prana* to "pierce" every atom of the body.

Maithuna: Ritual sexual intercourse in Tantric tradition of yoga.

Manipura chakra: The third chakra upward from the base of the spine. Region of the solar plexus. Center of energy.

Mantra: A sound (syllable, word, phrase) with spiritual meaning used in meditative practices.

Mantra yoga: A branch of yoga involving mantras and a study of inner vibrations.

Master: Equivalent to "esteemed teacher," or teacher of highest rank.

Matsyasana (Pose of a Fish): One of the backward-bending positions.

Mayurasana (Pose of a Peacock): One of the raised positions.

Meditation:

Intellectual—An intense act of reflection and pondering; the contemplation of subjects and ideas.

Transcendental—An act that involves the cessation of intellectual activities for the purpose of going beyond the intellect to reach a higher plane of consciousness.

Metaphysical teachings: Any teachings which are concerned with life beyond the physical, i.e., the spiritual dimension of existence. The term is used here to refer more specifically to Eastern philosophies of metaphysics.

Merudanda: Spinal column, "staff of life."

Manduka mudra: A special position of the tongue in which the tip of the tongue touches the soft palate. Also refers to a bodily pose known as the frog pose.

Mudras: Various techniques designed to tone up and stimulate aspects of the inner life of the body; also known as *bandhas.* *Mudra* also refers to traditional positions of the hands.

Mula bandha: Technique involving closing of the rectum to prevent escape of vital energy.

Muladara chakra: The first chakra, located at the base of the spine.

Nadis: In Indian thought, *nadis* are nervous-psychic channels of the subtle body, through which *prana* flows. They are 72,000 in number.

Natarajasana (Dancing Pose): One of the balancing exercises.

Nauli: Advanced technique involving contraction of the abdominal muscles; designed to stimulate and massage digestive organs.

Neti: Technique of cleaning nostrils with warm, salted water.

Nidra: One of the techniques of relaxation known as "sleepless sleep."

Om: In Indian thought, the most sacred sound of all the mantras. It is identified with divinity. In some schools of thought it is the primeval vibration signaling the beginning of the universe. There is a remarkable correspondence to this idea in the gospel of St. John, which begins with the sentence "In the beginning was the Word, and the Word was with God, and the Word was God."

Om breath: Breathing exercise in which the mantra *om* is silently pronounced during retention of breath.

Om ma ne pad me hum: The most famous Tibetan mantra and core of the Tibetan prayer wheel, meaning "Hail the Jewel (Grand Lama) in the Lotus Flower."

Padma asana (Pose of a Buddha—Lotus Pose): The most important sitting position in yoga.

Passimotasana: One of the forward-stretching poses.

Patanjali: An ancient sage and author of Yoga *sutras* expounding various aspects of yoga philosophy. He lived about 200 B.C.

Pavanamukasana: One of the bodily positions for improving digestion.

Pingala: In Indian thought, the nervous channel beginning in the right nostril; after criss-crossing with another channel *(ida)* which begins in the left nostril, *pingala* terminates at the base of the spine. Together with *shushumna, pingala* and *ida* are the three most important nervous-psychic channels of human makeup.

Plavini: One of the breathing techniques leading to the sensation of bodily lightness.

Prana: In Indian thought, a vital force in the breath; cosmic energy that animates all living creatures. Equivalent of *chi* and *ka*.

Prana-apana: Important mudra transforming cosmic energy in the breath *(prana)* into excretory energy of the body *(apana)*.

Pranayama: Breath control; a conscious interruption of natural breathing. *Pranayamas* are techniques to control the flow of cosmic energy into the system.

Pratyahara: A conscious withdrawal of sensory awareness to achieve a mental condition important in meditative practices.

Psyche: Greek word for "soul." The term is used here to correspond to that area of human nature which constitutes an inner life, including both soul and spirit.

Puraka: Inhalation in the practice of breath control.

Raja yoga: A branch of yoga philosophy dealing with mental and spiritual development that leads to the unfolding of higher powers and self-realization.

Rechaka: Exhalation in the practice of breath control.

Reincarnation: Literal rebirth, or "returning to flesh." Important doctrine in Eastern philosophies which teaches that one life is not enough to complete spiritual development of the individual so he is given a succession of lives to achieve it.

Salabhasana (Pose of a Locust): One of the backward-bending *asanas;* important for maintaining a supple spine.

Samadhi: The highest mental and spiritual state in yoga philosophy. A superconscious state of cosmic identification.

Samana: One of the vital energies or airs related to digestive powers.

Sarvangasana (Shoulder Stand): One of the inverted poses. After the headstand, it is considered the most powerful pose for its effect on the body. It tones up the nest of glands located in the throat.

Savasana: A classical supine pose of complete relaxation.

Self: The wholeness of the individual, which includes body, mind, soul, and spirit.

Shakti: An energy power often related to the female principle.

Shanmukhi mudra (Ten-fingered Gesture): Breathing exercise with special bodily posture that leads to stillness and revitalization of the five senses.

Shirshasana (Headstand): The most famous of all poses in physical yoga. Believed to have the greatest benefit of all poses.

Shitali: One of the breathing exercises for cooling, listed in an old treatise as a technique of longevity.

Shiva: In Indian thought, the symbol of creation; the male principle.

Shivasamhita: One of the classical treatises on Hatha yoga describing eighty-four *asanas,* or bodily postures.

Shushumna: A psychic channel inside the spinal cord; a passage for the raising of Kundalini power, as in Kundalini yoga.

Sidha asana (The Perfect or Auspicious Pose): One of the cross-legged positions used in meditative practices and breath control.

Siddhis: Higher powers of human makeup.

Simhasana (Pose of a Lion): Throat and face exercise considered a technique of longevity.

Soul: The personal manifestation of one's essential being; a complement to body and mind; the third dimension of one's existence, encompassing conscience and emotion.

Spirit: The impersonal spark of divinity within us that links us to cosmic divinity.

Sukhasana (Easy Pose): Simple cross-legged position.

Supta-vajrasana: One of the back-bending poses to limber up the small of the back, insteps, and knees.

Surya bhedana (Piercing of the Sun): A *pranayama* that involves inhaling through the right nostril.

Svadisthana chakra: The second chakra, or psychic center, related to sexual organs.

Swami: An honorable title in India, given during an initiation ceremony to a spiritually evolved yogi.

Tantra or Tantric yoga: Branch of yoga teaching reintegration through the act of sexual union.

Taoist yoga: Form of Chinese yoga embracing many ideas from Chinese philosophies. Many breath controls, meditative practices, and exercises designed for longevity.

Tibetan yoga: Modified version of Indian yoga including many mystical and magical rituals and dealing in part with life after physical expiration.

Trataka: An eye exercise for strengthening the eyesight by gazing.

Tutcheff, F. (1804–1873): A major poet of the golden age of Russian literature.

Uddiyan: Abdominal contraction—a powerful exercise to stimulate the digestive system.

Upanishads: The ancient Indian scriptures composed around 1200 B.C. containing the basic principles of the Hindu religion. Influenced the development of Indian yoga philosophy.

Ushtrasana (Pose of a Camel): One of the backward-bending *asanas.*

Vajroli mudra: An advanced technique for controlling movement of semen during the sexual act.

Vayus: Ten vital airs or energies. They are *prana* (breathing), *apana* (excretion), *samana* (digestion), *vyana* (circulation), *udana* (coughing), *naga* (eructation), *kurma* (blinking), *krikara* (sneezing), *dhanam-jaya* (assimilation), *deva-datta* (yawning).

Viparetha karani (Inverted Gesture, or Half Shoulder Stand): In some treatises, classified as a *mudra.*

Vishuddha chakra: The fifth chakra, located in the throat.

Yantra: Yoga of geometrical forms practiced in India, Tibet, and China.

Yin/yang: Male-female principle as represented in Chinese Taoist tradition.

Yoga: From the Sanskrit root *yuj*, which means "to link, unite, or join." The highest aim of yoga is a unification of the personal spirit with the universal spirit, a state of cosmic consciousness known as *samadhi.*

Yoga nidra: Technique for attaining complete rest, or "sleepless sleep of the yogi."

Yoga mudra: One of the classical *mudras* known as the symbol of yoga; it tones the whole body.

Yogi: One who practices yoga.

Yoni place: Area between anus and sexual organs.

Zen: A branch of Buddhism known as Ch'an in China; later introduced to Japan where it became widely known as Zen—a method of enlightenment which transcends intellect through the use of koans.

Index